— Healthy Cooking —

DIABETIC
COOKBOOK

Healthy Cooking

DIABETIC
COOKBOOK

Paul Morgan

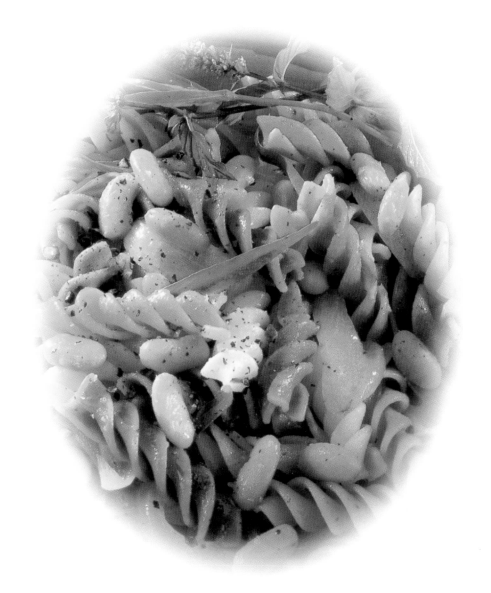

AN OCEANA BOOK

This edition published by Silverdale Books,
an imprint of Bookmart Ltd., in 2006

Bookmart Ltd.
Blaby Road
Wigston
Leicester
LE18 4SE

ISBN 1-84509-231-7

QUMHCDC

Manufactured in Singapore by
Pica Digital Pte. Ltd.
Printed in Singapore by
Star Standard Industries (Pte) Ltd

It is always sensible to consult your doctor before changing your diet
regime, but it is essential to do so if you suffer from any medical
condition or are taking medication of any kind. If you are concerned about
any symptoms that develop after changing your diet, consult your doctor
immediately. Information is given without any guarantees on the part of the
author and publisher, and they cannot be held responsible for the
contents of this book.

CONTENTS

INTRODUCTION

If you are reading this, it is likely that you have been diagnosed as a diabetic, or are worried – because of your family history, perhaps, or because you are concerned about your weight – that you might become one. And if you fall into the first category, you will not be alone: there are 1.8 million diabetics in Britain (3 per cent of the population, and an increase of 400,000 cases in just 8 years); and, in 2002, there were 13.3 million in the US (the number had risen from 5.8 million in 1980 and has almost certainly continued to rise). These figures show that it is far from unreasonable to be worried about developing diabetes, and the problems to which it leads, such as high blood pressure and heart disease.

So why is diabetes mellitus so prevalent nowadays? There are several answers, each of which interrelates with the others: first, obesity is becoming more and more common; second, modern technology means that many of us are less physically active than we should be; third, unhealthy 'fast food' and commercially processed foods are playing an increasing part in convenience lifestyles; and, fourth, established principles of healthy eating are either not taught to children or ignored by adults. Worryingly, too, it is becoming clear that the fast-food, inactive lifestyle of many children is making it more likely that they will develop diabetes later in life. This book is primarily concerned with the dietary measures you can take to control or avoid diabetes, however – and in essence, a healthy diet is, with certain changes in emphasis, a diabetic diet.

WHAT IS A HEALTHY DIET?

For 20 years or more, theories about what constitutes a healthy diet have chopped and changed. First, all fat was considered to be bad for you – then it was found that some types of fat can protect your heart. Then butter was considered bad, while margarine was thought to be good for you – but after a while, scientists discovered that margarine contained substances called trans fatty acids, which are extremely bad for you. At the same time, all cholesterol was once considered dangerous, but now we know that one type of cholesterol is, in fact, very good for you. Then scientists devised the

A WORD OF WARNING

If you have been diagnosed as a diabetic and take insulin or other drugs to control your condition, you should have received dietary and lifestyle advice from your doctor and, ideally, a dietician – if you have not, consult your doctor as soon as possible.

But you should also consult your doctor before making any major changes to your diet or starting an exercise programme. The reason is that the measures you take will probably reduce your blood sugar levels and necessitate a change in your drug treatment, which was already reducing and stabilizing these levels, because very low blood sugar levels (hypoglycaemia) can be extremely dangerous, leading to coma. Your doctor may wish to monitor your levels until it is clear what effect your new regime is having.

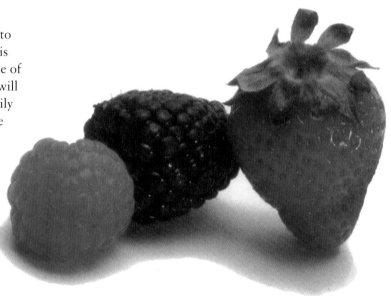

Try to get into the habit of eating healthy snacks, for example fruit and nuts, instead of biscuits and crisps.

glycaemic index, which rates carbohydrates according to how quickly they affect blood sugar levels, and helps us differentiate between the various different forms of carbohydrate.

You could be forgiven for being confused. But now, after years of research, scientists have a fairly clear picture of the effects of nutrition on our health. It is beyond question that by avoiding certain foods and eating others you can significantly reduce your chances of developing diabetes (and, thereby, heart disease and other problems) and improve your chances in the long term if you are already affected by it.

This book will show you how to do just that. First, we will look at what diabetes is and what causes it, and show how the make-up of some foods can lead to a condition called insulin resistance, the precursor of diabetes. Then we will examine how healthy eating can reduce your chances of developing heart disease, which often develops alongside insulin resistance. And then you can choose from a range of mouth-watering, diabetic-friendly recipes. It may be a cliché, but like many clichés it is true: when it comes to your health, you really are what you eat!

WHAT IS DIABETES?

Sugar, which fuels the cells of your body, is carried in your bloodstream in the form of a basic sugar called glucose – all the forms of sugar and all the carbohydrates that you eat are broken down into simpler forms of sugar and then glucose during the digestive process. The level of glucose in your blood relates to the amount of such foods in your diet, but is controlled by insulin, a hormone produced in the pancreas. This promotes the uptake of glucose by individual cells and also its storage in the liver and fat cells. If there is insufficient or no insulin, or if the insulin that is produced does not do its job properly, the level of glucose in the blood will become abnormally high.

This may sound innocuous, but it is far from it. The cells' inability to receive glucose causes hunger, weight loss and tiredness. Importantly, though, high blood glucose levels not only damage the kidneys, so that waste products of the body's chemical processes are not properly filtered out of the blood and into the urine, but also damage nerves and blood vessels – the result is a rise in blood pressure, which is a major risk factor in heart disease.

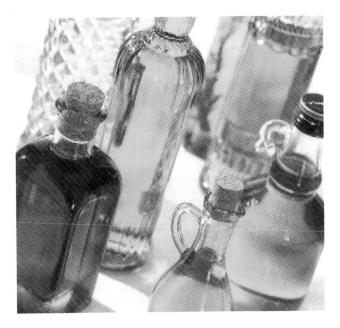

Choosing olive oil as your main source of dietary fat, combined with eating a healthy diet, can help reduce your risk of cardiovascular disease and diabetes.

Types of diabetes

The are two main types of diabetes mellitus: type 1, also known as insulin-dependent diabetes (IDDM); and type 2, also known as non-insulin-dependent diabetes (NIDDM). In IDDM, which usually develops in early life between the ages of 10 and 16, no insulin is produced by the body and regular insulin injections are required (though soon it may be possible to inhale insulin), as well as dietary measures. The cause is an abnormal (autoimmune) defensive reaction by the body, often following a viral infection, to the insulin-producing cells.

NIDDM usually appears later in life, building up gradually after the 40s – there may be no symptoms for many years, but blood tests can show the presence of an early form of the condition called pre-diabetes. In NIDDM either too little insulin is produced, or the insulin that is produced is ineffective. In most cases, insulin need not be given and the condition can be controlled by dietary and lifestyle measures and medication. NIDMM can also develop during pregnancy (gestational diabetes), though this is often detected during screening; it usually resolves itself after the birth, but makes it more likely that diabetes will develop later in life.

Insulin resistance and 'syndrome X'

If you are overweight (see box on page 11) and inactive and frequently eat carbohydrates that boost your blood sugar levels quickly (and especially if you have a hereditary predisposition to diabetes) you are likely to develop insulin resistance: insulin starts to lose the ability to make cells take up glucose. As a result, the levels of both insulin and sugar in your blood are always higher than they should be. Even though there may be no symptoms, insulin resistance causes pre-diabetes, which usually leads to full-blown diabetes within 10 years – unless the excess weight is lost and dietary measures are taken.

In many cases, people with insulin resistance have 'syndrome X'. This is a condition in which there are high levels of fats, glucose and insulin in the blood, but low levels of 'good' cholesterol (see page 12) – together, these lead to high blood pressure and are a major risk for developing heart disease.

The bottom line

Where necessary, diabetes is treated by either insulin or other medication. But other measures are needed to cope with diabetes and its associated heart problems – and these can also help prevent insulin resistance from turning into diabetes. If you are diabetic, it is vital that you follow the specific diet that your doctor has prescribed for you – the dishes in this book are all diabetic-friendly, though some more so than others. If you suspect that you have insulin resistance, consult your doctor. But if you just want to reduce the risk of developing insulin resistance, diabetes or heart problems, you should follow these rules (though introduce dietary and lifestyle changes gradually, so that your blood sugar levels are lowered at a moderate rate):
- eat small meals regularly, never missing one
- plan your meals around wholegrain foods, such as wholegrain breads and cereals, potatoes with their skins on, rice and pasta
- lower your intake of calories if you are overweight and increase physical activity, then maintain your weight at a healthy level
- reduce salt levels in your diet
- avoid table sugar and sugary foods
- choose foods that have a low glycaemic index (see page 10)
- reduce your intake of saturated fats and trans fats (see page 12) and choose unsaturated fats instead

- reduce your intake of dairy foods and use low-fat alternatives
- eat five helpings of fruit and vegetables a day
- use fresh or frozen foods rather than processed ones
- drink only moderate amounts of alcohol
- avoid commercial 'diabetic foods', which are often high in fat and calories.

The overall aim is to keep blood sugar levels moderate and stable, to lose weight and to prevent damage to the cardiovascular system. Over the next few pages we will explain the significance of the rules and show how to put the theory into practice.

ARE YOU AT RISK?

There are often few symptoms if you are developing diabetes, nor are there any symptoms of the high blood pressure, known as 'the silent killer', that it causes. But while it is important to check your blood pressure regularly it also is important, if you are at risk, to have a blood test to see if you are developing diabetes or are insulin resistant and pre-diabetic.

Discuss taking a test with your doctor if you fall into one of these risk categories:

- you are obese, and especially if you carry too much weight on your stomach
- you have a family history of diabetes
- you are of Asian or Afro-Caribbean origin
- you have had gestational diabetes
- you have given birth to a large baby.

CARBOHYDRATES

Many people associate diabetes primarily with eating too much sugar. They are correct, but it is not just table sugar and obviously sugary foods that are the problem. Carbohydrates are the body's primary source of fuel and are an essential part of a healthy diet. But there are three types of carbohydrate: sugars, fibre, and starch, and all of them are built from molecules of sugar. Until fairly recently, they used to be described as 'complex' or 'simple' carbohydrates, depending on whether they were simple forms of sugar or consisted of linked forms of sugar, and it was believed that simple carbohydrates should be avoided and complex ones preferred.

YOU SHOULD ALSO CONSULT YOUR DOCTOR IF YOU HAVE THESE SYMPTOMS OF DIABETES:

- you are becoming thirstier
- you urinate more often
- you are starting to tire more easily
- you have lost a lot of weight
- your vision is sometimes blurred
- you have genital itching or recurring infections of thrush

People often put symptoms such as these down to being overworked, or just to growing older. It may be that factors such as these are responsible, but it is important to rule out diabetes as a cause.

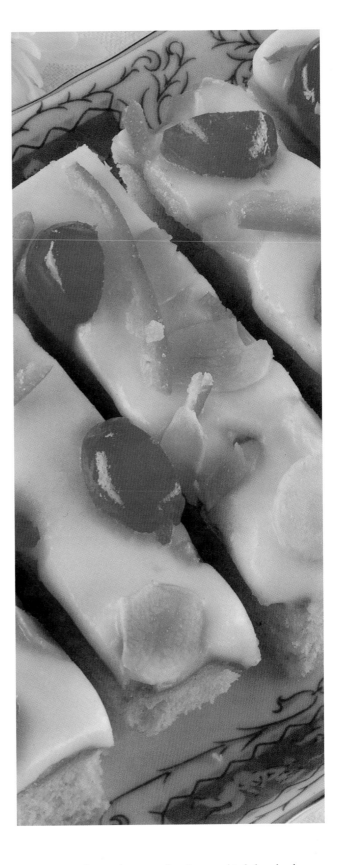

Try to avoid any desserts that have a high level of sugar or saturated fat, for example cakes and biscuits.

THE GLYCAEMIC INDEX

Today this categorization is no longer used. Instead, nutritionists classify carbohydrates according to their glycaemic index value. During the digestive process, carbohydrates are broken down into the simplest forms of sugar, and the glycaemic index (GI) measures how quickly this happens with individual foods and so how fast levels of sugar in the blood rise – a high glycaemic index value means that the carbohydrate raises them very quickly. Eating a preponderance of high glycaemic index foods makes it more likely that you will develop insulin resistance, high blood pressure and, eventually, diabetes.

High or low?

In essence, whether a food has a high or low glycaemic index depends on how quickly its carbohydrates are converted to simple sugar during the digestive process. Foods that have not been processed – whole-grain foods – still contain their original fibre, which slows down the rate at which carbohydrates are converted to simple sugars and so also slows down the rate at which sugar enters the bloodstream. However, the type of starch in the food is important, too: potatoes, for example, contain a starch that is broken down quickly during digestion. Other factors affecting the GI value are: ripeness – ripe fruit has a higher GI than unripe fruit; acidity – vinegar and lemon juice delay stomach emptying and so reduce the GI value; and the size of food particles – small particles are more easily absorbed and increase the GI value.

Low GI foods include soy, beans, fruit, milk, grainy bread and oats; medium ones include orange juice, sugar and wholemeal bread; while high GI foods include alcohol, mashed potatoes, sugar, small-grain rice and white bread. It might seem a daunting prospect to exist solely on low GI foods, but it is not necessary to do so. Luckily, however, eating a low GI food reduces the GI value of high GI foods when they are eaten at the same time – if you eat cornflakes (high GI) with milk (low GI) your blood sugar levels will not go up as quickly – what is known as the 'glycaemic load' is reduced. So if you plan your menus with caution you can still eat some high GI foods.

Remember, though, that if you have eaten any sugary foods – cakes, biscuits and pastries, for example – you should reduce your intake of carbohydrates, whatever their glycaemic index, to compensate.

CHECK THE LABEL

Food labels can be misleading, so it is important to read them carefully. Phrases such as 'made with wheat flour' do not necessarily mean that the product is a whole-grain food. To be sure that it is, look for a main ingredient that is specifically described as being 'whole-grain'.

Another problem with food labels is that they do not always give the amount of sugar that a product contains. In particular, you should be wary of 'low-fat' products, which often contain surprisingly high levels of sugar. The best solution is to rely on fresh, unprocessed food.

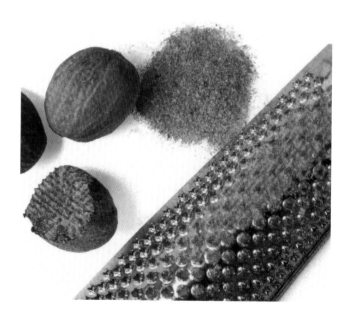

Many people believe that their food will be insipid if they cut down on salt, but this is not true. As an alternative try using herbs, lemon juice, vinegar or spices like nutmeg to add that extra bit of flavour.

FOODS TO CHOOSE

(Low glycaemic index carbohydrates)

Bran and *porridge oats*

Barley, *buckwheat*, and *bulgur wheat*

Some fruits – apples, citrus, berries, peaches, pears, plums and rhubarb

Pasta

Some vegetables – avocados, aubergines, beans (runner and green), broccoli, cabbage, cauliflower, carrots, celery, courgette, cucumber, leeks, onions, lettuce, mushrooms, olives, peas, peppers, spinach and tomatoes

---

FOODS TO USE

(Medium glycaemic index carbohydrates)

Pure wheat cereals

Granary and *whole-wheat bread*

Basmati or *long-grained rice*, *wild rice* and *couscous*

Corn – cornmeal, corn oil, sweetcorn

Some fruits – apricots, bananas, melon, dried fruit, pineapples and mangos

Vegetables – new potatoes, sweet potatoes, beetroot and artichokes

---

FOODS TO AVOID

(High glycaemic index carbohydrates)

Breakfast cereals – cornflakes and sugar-coated cereals

White bread, *cakes, biscuits, bagels, buns, muffins, pancakes* and *doughnuts*

White and *brown rice*

Some fruits – dates, prunes and watermelon

Gnocchi

Some vegetables – broad beans, potatoes (when mashed, baked, fried or roasted), parsnips and swede

Sugar – table, glucose, treacle and molasses

Tomato ketchup

THE DANGERS OF BEING OVERWEIGHT

Being overweight brings with the dangers of many health problems, but if you carry the extra pounds on your waist – in the classic 'beer belly' – you are far more at risk of developing diabetes and heart disease.

In fact, men with waists of more than 101 cm (40 in) and women with waists of more than 89 cm (35 in) are at between double and quadruple the risk of developing them. The reason is that fat that is stored around the stomach secretes hormones that play havoc with the production of insulin. As a result insulin resistance develops, leading to diabetes, high blood pressure and high cholesterol levels.

But if you are overweight, all is not lost. A reduction in your weight of 10 kg (22 lb) can significantly lower your chances of dying from diabetes and significantly reduce your blood pressure, blood glucose levels, blood fat levels, and blood 'bad' cholesterol levels; it can also increase your 'good' cholesterol levels.

FATS AND CHOLESTEROL

One of the dangers of insulin resistance and diabetes is that they both lead to heart disease, unless dietary measures are taken. So it is even more important than usual for people affected by these conditions to control their cholesterol levels.

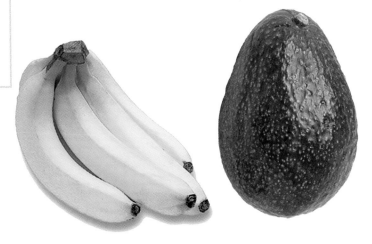

Bananas and avocados are both rich in potassium, which helps counteract the effect of too much salt.

For many years, scientists believed that the cholesterol that you eat is the villain of the piece when it comes to heart disease. In fact, about 75 per cent of the cholesterol in your blood is manufactured by your liver, while only 25 per cent of it is in your diet. And the liver uses dietary fat to make cholesterol. When this was appreciated, the emphasis moved to eating a low-fat and low-cholesterol diet. But then it was discovered that it is not only the amount of fat in your diet that is important, but how much of which type of fat you eat – and there are three main types of fat: saturated fats, unsaturated fats and trans fats.

Saturated fats are found in meat, poultry, lard and whole-milk dairy products, such as cheese, milk, butter and cream, but high levels are also found in some vegetable oils, such as coconut and palm oil.

Unsaturated fats, which typically are liquid at room temperature, are found in plant and vegetable oils, such as olive, peanut, sesame, safflower, corn, sunflower, canola, and soybean oil, and in avocados, oily fish (in the form of omega–3 fatty acid), and nuts and seeds.

Trans fats are man-made – a by-product of heating vegetable oils in the presence of hydrogen (which is why they are often referred to as 'hydrogenated vegetable oils' on product labels). They are found in commercially-baked goods, such as biscuits, snack foods, processed foods and commercially prepared fried foods, such as crisps. Some margarines also contain high levels of trans fats, especially brands that are 'hard' margarines – spreadable ones have less high levels as they are less hydrogenated (hydrogenation makes the fat hard at room temperature).

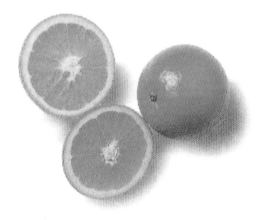

To many people the uses for citrus fruits extend only to drinks and to a few familiar dishes, but in reality their uses are practically limitless.

Where cholesterol comes in

Your body needs cholesterol to function correctly – it is involved in the production of hormones, the body's chemical messengers, as well as bile and vitamin D, and is found in every part of the body. For this reason, it is manufactured in the liver – and the liver uses fats to make it. If you eat too much saturated fat, the liver produces too much cholesterol. And, unfortunately, cholesterol is a soft, waxy substance that can stick to the lining of blood vessels and obstruct them if there are high levels of it in the blood.

As we have seen, liver-produced cholesterol, and so the cholesterol that is ultimately the result of fat consumption, accounts for around 75 per cent of the cholesterol found in your blood. The remaining 25 per cent comes from the cholesterol you eat. Dietary cholesterol is found in eggs, dairy products, meat, poultry, fish and shellfish, but the highest levels are found in egg yolks, meats such as liver and kidneys and shellfish. People who are diabetic or insulin resistant should monitor their cholesterol intake closely because of their increased risk of heart disease – vegetables, fruits, nuts, grains and cereals contain no cholesterol.

'Good' and 'bad' cholesterol

Cholesterol is carried around the body by chemicals called lipoproteins. There are two types: low-density lipoprotein (LDL) and high-density lipoprotein (HDL). If there is too much of the cholesterol carried by LDL, known as 'bad' cholesterol, plaque builds up on arterial walls. But HDL carries cholesterol away from the arteries to the liver, which breaks it down so that it can be excreted from the body; for this reason, HDL cholesterol is said to be 'good' cholesterol.

For some years, scientists have known that saturated fats, and, in particular, trans fats, increase the blood levels of harmful LDL cholesterol and lower levels of beneficial HDL cholesterol, while unsaturated fats have the opposite effect. In January 2005, however, researchers at the Dana-Farber Cancer Institute, in the US, reported that they had discovered the mechanism responsible. It appears that saturated fats trigger a biochemical activator in the liver that boosts LDL cholesterol production.

To sum up, then, a healthy-diabetic, healthy-heart diet is one that has low levels of saturated and trans fats, high levels of unsaturated fats and controlled levels of dietary cholesterol.

FOODS TO USE RARELY

(Rich in dietary cholesterol)
Organ meats – liver and kidneys
Eggs (especially ones from battery-farmed chickens)
Shellfish
Red meat

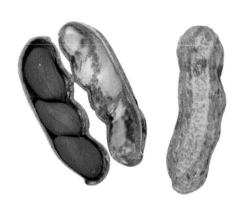

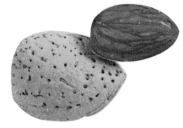

Besides tasting so good, nuts are an excellent source of protein as well as the B vitamins, vitamin E and minerals such as iron, calcium, magnesium and potassium.

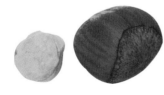

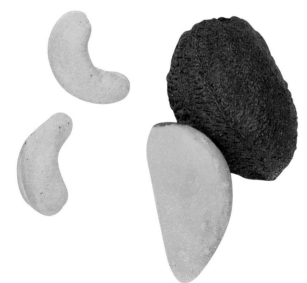

FOODS TO CHOOSE

(Containing unsaturated fat)
Vegetable oils – pure olive, peanut, walnut, sesame, corn, soybean, sunflower and safflower oils
Avocados
Oily fish – salmon, mackerel, tuna, herrings and so on
Nuts and *seeds*
Spreadable, unsaturated margarine

FOODS TO USE SPARINGLY

(Containing saturated fat)
Whole-fat milk (skimmed milk is preferable)
Butter, cream, cheese, full-fat yoghurt (low-fat is preferable), *ice cream*
Meat – beef, lamb and pork
Poultry – battery-farmed chicken (free-range is preferable), goose, duck and turkey (wild game, such as rabbit, wild duck and venison is better)
Lard
Eggs (especially ones from battery-farmed chickens)
Coconut oil and *palm oil*

FOODS TO AVOID

(Containing trans fat)
Ready-made commercial foods – cakes, biscuits and snack foods
Processed foods – sausages, pâté, scotch eggs, pies and so on
Commercially prepared fried foods – crisps, battered fish and chips
Hard margarine

SALT

The more salt you eat, the more your body retains fluid, and the more fluid there is, the harder your heart has to work to pump blood around your body. And the result of this increase in the heart's work rate is high blood pressure and the risk, over time, of developing heart failure. Some groups of people are said to be 'salt sensitive', and are at particular risk of heart damage even without a rise in blood pressure. They include the elderly, Afro-Caribbeans – and diabetics.

Doctors recommend that our daily intake of salt should be less than 6 grams – about a teaspoonful. This is especially important in the case of people who have insulin resistance or are diabetics, and so who may have nascent heart problems.

Hidden salt

The 6 gram target sounds an easy enough one to achieve, but in fact it is a very tall order. The reason is that this target refers to our total salt intake, not just to the salt that we add to our food, and there is a considerable amount of salt hidden in the foods many of us eat. Processed foods are mainly to blame – in fact, researchers estimate that around 75 per cent of our salt intake comes from them.

It is obvious that some foods contain high salt levels: salted nuts, crisps, olives and anchovies, for example, all taste and are salty. But bacon, cheese, pickles, stock cubes, sausages and smoked meat and fish contain salt, too. And some brands of biscuits, pizzas, 'ready meals', soups and breakfast cereals are also surprisingly high in salt.

The only way to check which processed foods are high in salt is to read product labels carefully. It is easy to come unstuck when you do this, however, because some labels do not refer to the product's salt content but to its sodium content (salt is made up of sodium and chloride). The two values are not the same – in fact, you have to multiply the sodium value by 2.5 to obtain the real salt content.

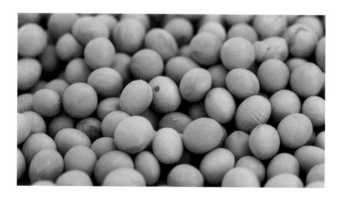

It is hard to think of any other common, widely used foodstuff that provides as many benefits as the soya bean. The nutritional advantages that soy can provide are numerous. It is the most complete form of high-quality vegetable protein available, and is high in essential amino acids, especially lysine, which makes it very similar to animal proteins such as meat and eggs.

Reducing your salt intake

If you cut down on salt, your blood pressure will fall within weeks, even if it was not too high in the first place. And that means that your risk of developing heart disease or having a stroke will also fall.

Many people think that their food will lack taste if they cut down on salt, but this is a myth. You may find that your diet is a little bland for the first week or so, but your taste buds soon adapt. Adopt these salt reduction strategies and you will find the process much more easy.

AVOID PROCESSED FOODS

Check the salt levels of all commercially prepared foods, including everyday products such as bread
- Throw away your salt shaker
- Make your own salt-free stocks and sauces
- Use alternative seasonings, such as lemon juice, herbs and vinegar
- Eat fresh fruit (bananas and avocados in particular) and vegetables: the potassium they contain helps counter the effect of dietary salt
- Do not switch to sea salt, rock salt, or garlic salt – they are not different to normal salt
- Ask your doctor whether salt substitutes are suitable for you.

FOODS TO AVOID
All types of salt – table, rock, sea and garlic
Obviously salty foods – anchovies, salted nuts and ready-salted potato chips

FOODS TO USE SPARINGLY
(High in salt)
Commercially made foods – biscuits, supermarket bread, cheese biscuits and crisps
Ready-made meals – including pasta, pizzas, curries and Asian cuisine
Tinned foods – baked beans, spaghetti, meats and vegetables
Preserved and smoked foods – bacon, ham, pickles, spiced sausage, stock cubes and sauces

---

CALCULATE YOUR SALT INTAKE

If you must eat processed foods – and it can be hard not to – try to make sure that you stay within the recommended daily intake of 6 grams of salt. Read a product's label to find the number of grams of salt in 100 grams of the contents. If the quantity of sodium is given, multiply by 2.5 to calculate the actual salt content. (If the value is given in milligrams, or 'mg', divide by 1,000 to convert it to grams.)

Then look for the total weight of the contents, or estimate the proportion of them that you intend to use. Divide the weight that you will use by 100, then multiply by the number of grams of salt in each 100 grams and you will discover how much salt you will eat. The results can be surprising: one small (200 g) tin of baked beans can contain as much as 1.7 grams of salt – just under a third of your total recommended intake; one slice of white, refined bread contains 0.61 grams of salt – so just the bread making up a lunchtime sandwich could well account for just under a fifth of your total recommended daily intake.

For those people who follow a healthy diet, fresh summer fruits are most certainly considered nutrient-rich foods. There are many things inside fresh fruits and vegetables that make them highly beneficial. They provide an array of vitamins, potassium and dietary fibre in addition to important phytonutrients that are thought to protect against cancer, heart disease and other diseases associated with ageing.

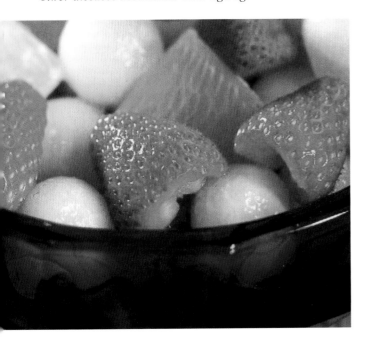

SALT SUBSTITUTES

Some people find that their food tastes a little bland when they switch to a low-salt diet, and even though their taste buds will adapt within a few weeks some people find that they need a little help to make the change. A number of salt substitutes are on the market, but these contain part sodium and part potassium and in certain circumstances it is possible to overload your body with potassium – consult your doctor before using a commercial salt substitute.

Make your own

This recipe for a salt substitute relies on the principle that a sour flavour is a good substitute for a salty one. It uses the grapefruit peel (or lemon or orange peel, for a weaker taste) and citric acid crystal. Also known as 'sour salt' and 'lemon salt', these can be found in the baking section of supermarkets or in delicatessens.

Ingredients
- the peel of 1 grapefruit
- 1 tbsp ground allspice
- $1/2$ tbsp citric acid crystals

Makes 3 tablespoons

Method

1 Peel the grapefruit as thinly as possible, then scrape away all the white parts. Dry the peel overnight near a source of heat.

2 Grind the dried peel in a coffee grinder or spice grinder, then combine it with the other ingredients. Put the mixture into a well-sealed bottle and shake well to mix. Store in a dry place.

Variations

Add a tablespoon of freshly ground black pepper to the mixture to make it into citrus pepper, an ideal seasoning for meat.

PROTEIN

Protein, made up from chemicals called amino acids, makes up the building blocks of all our body's tissues except stored fat. You need to eat a certain amount of protein every day – a minimum of one gram for every kilogram of body weight – to prevent the body from starting to break down tissue. And you need more than that if you want to build up healthy muscles and robust bones.

But the quantity of protein you eat is not the whole story. What is important is that you eat a variety of amino acids, which means protein from a variety of sources. This does not mean that it is essential to eat steaks, for example, because you can obtain a full range of proteins from vegetable and fruit sources, if you are a vegetarian. Variety is the watchword.

Protective protein?

Scientists have theorized that eating large amounts of protein might have beneficial effects on the cardiovascular system, but the question has not yet been resolved. However, one large-scale, 14-year study – the Nurses' Health Study, in the US – showed that women who ate about 110 grams of protein a day were 25 per cent less likely to suffer from heart problems than women who ate 68 grams a day; whether the protein came from animal or vegetable sources did not

matter, and nor did the fat levels in the women's diet. So there are certainly no dangers to eating relatively large amounts of protein, though preferably from sources that do not contain saturated fats, and there may be a beneficial effect.

One protein that has definitely been shown to help prevent heart disease by lowering cholesterol levels is soy. An analysis of 38 different trials has shown that eating 50 grams of soy protein a day instead of animal protein lowered LDL cholesterol levels by 12.9 per cent – a significant figure.

FOODS TO CHOOSE

(*'Good' protein – lower in saturated fats*)
Vegetables – beans, brown rice, lentils, millet and pulses
Soybeans
Nuts – brazil, peanuts and pinenuts
Seeds – sesame
Free-range chicken and *turkey* (but remove the skin)
Locally sourced lean cuts of non-intensively reared meats – beef, lamb, pork and veal
Free-range chicken eggs (but not duck or goose eggs)

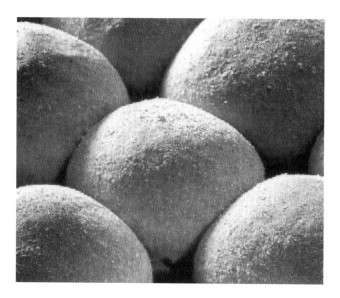

Whole-wheat bread or rolls are high in insoluble fibre. This type of fibre creates a feeling of fullness in the stomach, and its water-holding quality helps to create bulk and moisture in the bowels.

FIBRE

Our bodies cannot digest some of the food that we eat, and it is this indigestible material that is known as dietary fibre. Most people know that a diet high in fibre is good for your bowel function and can protect against disorders of the intestines, such as cancer of the colon, but it is less well known that fibre can also lower the levels of cholesterol in your blood – and, as we have seen, it is vital that diabetics, who are at greatly increased risk of developing heart disease, should do all that they can to control the levels of cholesterol in their blood.

There are two types of fibre: insoluble and soluble (the latter is so-called because it forms a gel when mixed with liquid). Insoluble fibre plays the main part in promoting bowel function, and high levels of it are found in foods such as whole-wheat bread, wheat cereals, rice, barley, grains, cabbage, carrots and so on.

But it is soluble fibre that reduces blood cholesterol – though it is not clear how it does this. It is found in oats, oat bran, oatmeal, peas, beans, barley and fruits.

Five a day

So it makes sense to increase your intake of foods rich in fibre, and especially of those rich in soluble fibre – generally, it is recommended that you should eat five portions of fibre-rich fruit and vegetables a day. And, of course, foods such as these are low in saturated fats and cholesterol. Make sure that you read labels carefully, though, because some commercial, processed products that claim to be rich in fibre in fact contain very little of it.

VITAMINS, MINERALS AND ANTIOXIDANTS

There is absolutely no doubt that every one of our body's systems needs vitamins and minerals to function, and the cardiovascular system, which is put under particular pressure by diabetes, is no exception. Vitamins act as catalysts, initiating and controlling chemical reactions in the body. Only small amounts of them are needed – they are known as micronutrients – and they must be obtained from our diet, because the body cannot manufacture them. If you follow the rules for healthy eating given in this book, and take a multivitamin supplement every day, as a precaution, you should absorb all the vitamins and minerals that your body requires. But sometimes the way that we treat and cook food reduces its content of micronutrients. Follow these rules to make sure that you can meet your body's requirements.

Avoid processed foods, and canned foods in particular, because these can be surprisingly low in vitamin content.

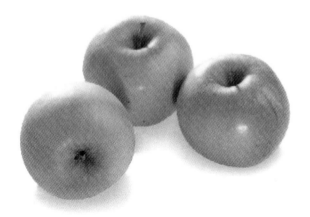

Use the skin of fruit and vegetables where possible – instead of peeling, wash and scrub them.

FOODS TO CHOOSE

(High in soluble fibre)

Oatmeal and *oat bran*

Lentils, beans and *peas*

Apples, bananas, blueberries, oranges, pears and *strawberries*

Sweetcorn, spinach, spring greens and *broccoli*

Nuts – almonds, brazil, hazel, peanuts, pecan, pistachio and walnuts

Seeds – sesame, sunflower and pumpkin

FOODS TO USE

(High in insoluble fibre)

Whole grains – bran, wheat, couscous, brown rice, bulgur and barley

Wholewheat and *granary bread*

Wholewheat pasta

Wholewheat flour

Wholegrain breakfast cereals

Fruit – both fresh and dried

All vegetables – but especially brussels sprouts, carrots, cabbage, okra, parsnips, sweetcorn, courgette, cucumber, celery, tomatoes and unpeeled potatoes

Always use fresh or frozen fruit and vegetables, because vitamin levels decrease as these foods age. It is not generally realized that freezing preserves vitamin content, but chilling fruit and vegetables in a refrigerator before heating them can reduce levels of vitamins such as vitamin C and folic acid by up to 30 per cent. Remember that frozen vegetables – peas, especially – are often more vitamin-rich than fresh ones, because they are frozen a very short time after being picked.

Keep all foods away from heat, light and air, all of which reduce levels of vitamin C and the B vitamins. Store vegetables in airtight bags.

Use the skin of fruits and vegetables wherever possible and avoid trimming them too much. Instead of peeling, wash or scrub them – most of the nutritional value of fruits and vegetables is contained in the skin or the area underneath it.

Keep the water you have used to cook vegetables and use it as a base for stock or sauces – otherwise you will lose the valuable vitamins and minerals that have leached into the water.

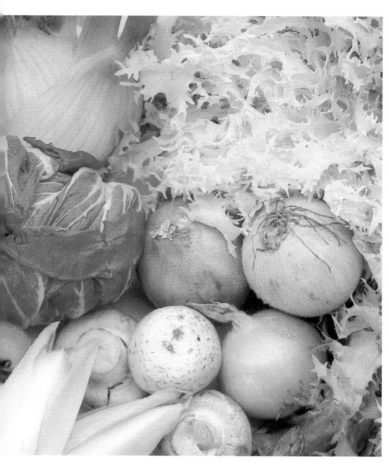

A fresh vegetable salad is far more beneficial in terms of nutritional value than cooked vegetables. Try to find ways to enjoy fresh flavours of vegetables in an assortment of recipes.

Take a daily multivitamin supplement – it can be hard to obtain sufficient quantities of some vitamins, such as B12 and folic acid from your diet; and fibre-rich foods contain chemicals called phytates, which can bind with some minerals and interfere with their absorption. But think of it as a nutritional safety net, rather than as a substitute for healthy eating.

HOMOCYSTEINE

Some research has linked high levels of a protein called homocysteine in the blood with high levels of the 'bad', plaque-causing LDL cholesterol – these present a risk to everybody, but the risk is especially high in the case of diabetics. The theory is that homocysteine changes cholesterol into this 'bad' form. Normally, homocysteine is broken down to form new proteins for the body with the help of vitamins B6 and B12 and folic acid, and it is thought that people with high

homocysteine levels may lack sufficient of these vitamins in their diet.

Research has yet to confirm this theory, though several studies are ongoing and more should be known soon. Until the results are in, however, it would be sensible to make sure that you eat sufficient vitamin B6 and B12 and folic acid in your diet. Foods rich in them include asparagus, avocados, bananas, beans, cabbage, carrots, fish, lentils and spinach, and – though these should be eaten sparingly – cheese, milk, beef, yoghurt and eggs.

ANTIOXIDANTS

Many of our bodily structures can be damaged by the presence of what are known as 'free radicals' – technically speaking, these are atoms that have unpaired electrons. The most common free radical is radical oxygen, which can damage cells and increase the likelihood that LDL 'bad' cholesterol forms fatty plaques in arteries – again, a major risk for people with diabetes or pre-diabetes.

When this was realised, in the 1990s, nutritionists started to look at the antioxidants, which combat radical oxygen – the most common ones being vitamins C and E and beta-carotene (a precursor to vitamin A), and lycopene. Soon antioxidant supplements became increasingly popular, and today some 30 per cent of Americans take them. Unfortunately, they do not reduce the risks of heart disease or stroke, as a series of studies, and meta-studies (that is, studies of studies), have shown.

Nevertheless, it has been shown that a diet that is high in antioxidants is protective against heart disease. The answer to this conundrum is thought to be that in practice the effect of dietary antioxidants relies on the interaction between the antioxidants and other dietary ingredients: minerals, perhaps, or fibre. So it is important to eat a diet rich in antioxidants – that means richly coloured fruit and vegetables that contain chemicals called flavonoids, such as apricots, blueberries, bilberries, broccoli, carrots, mangos, peppers and spinach, and, in particular, tomatoes (though these should be cooked to release maximum quantities of flavonoids). And, just to show that a healthy diet need not be without its luxuries, there are high levels of flavonoids in both dark chocolate and red wine – though both should be enjoyed in moderation.

VITAMIN- AND MINERAL-RICH FOODS

(NB Pre-menopausal women and women taking HRT should eat more of foods containing vitamins that are depleted by the female hormone oestrogen.)

Vitamin A (antioxidant)

Retinol: butter, cod liver oil, cheese and beta-carotene: apricots, cantaloupe, carrots, kale, peach, peas, spinach and sweet potatoes

Vitamin B1

Beans, brown rice, milk, oatmeal, vegetables, whole grains and yeast (depleted by alcohol, caffeine, exposure to air and water, food additives and oestrogen)

Vitamin B2

Eggs, fish, meat, milk, vegetables, and whole grains (depleted by alcohol, caffeine, oestrogen and zinc)

Vitamin B3

Avocado, eggs, fish, meat, peanuts, prunes, seeds and whole grains (destroyed by canning and some sleeping pills; depleted by alcohol and oestrogen)

Vitamin B5

Bran, eggs, green vegetables, meat, whole grains and yeast (destroyed by canning)

Vitamin B6

Avocado, bananas, cabbage, cantaloupe, fish, milk, eggs, seeds and wheat bran (destroyed by alcohol, heat, oestrogen and processing techniques during production of commercial food)

Vitamin B folic acid

Apricots, avocados, beans, carrots, green vegetables, melons, oranges and whole wheat (destroyed by commercial food processing techniques, cooking and exposure to water and air, depleted by alcohol)

Vitamin B12

Dairy products, fish and meat (depleted by alcohol, exposure to sunlight and water, oestrogen and sleeping tablets)

Vitamin C (antioxidant)

Broccoli, cabbage, cauliflower, citrus fruits, green peppers, spinach, tomatoes and potatoes (destroyed by boiling, exposure to air, and carbon dioxide and long storage; depleted by alcohol, aspirin, oestrogen, stress and tobacco)

Vitamin D

Cod liver oil, dairy products and oily fish (depleted by lack of sunlight)

Vitamin E (antioxidant)

Almonds, broccoli, eggs, kale, oats, olive oil, peanuts, soybeans, seeds, spinach and wheat germ (destroyed by commercial food processing techniques, freezing, heat, oxygen and chlorine; depleted by smoking and use of contraceptive pills)

Vitamin K

Broccoli, cod liver oil, eggs, green vegetables, live yoghurt, tomatoes and whole grains

Magnesium

Bitter chocolate, brown rice, nuts, soybeans and whole wheat (depleted by caffeine and stress)

Zinc (antioxidant)

Eggs, meat, mushrooms, yeast and whole grains (inhibited by caffeine and smoking)

Potassium

Avocados, bananas, dried fruit, green vegetables, nuts and potatoes (lost in diarrhoea and sweat)

Selenium (antioxidant)

Broccoli, onions, tomatoes, tuna and wheat germ

TOO MUCH CAN BE DANGEROUS

Many people take high doses of vitamin supplements, without having taken medical advice. But doing so can be dangerous, because in many cases the effects of high doses are not known, and in some cases the effects have been confirmed to be dangerous. For example, it was once thought that very high doses of vitamin E might help prevent heart disease, but several studies have failed to show this and a recent study suggests that they may make heart failure more likely. And the list goes on: too much calcium can lead to lethargy, confusion and coma; excess vitamin B6 can cause a nerve disorder that leads to loss of feeling in the arms and legs; high doses of vitamin A can increase the risk of cardiovascular disease – a major risk for diabetics – and can damage your liver; excessive doses of vitamin C can cause abdominal pain, nausea and diarrhoea; and so on.

The message is clear: do not take high-dose vitamin supplements unless they have been prescribed by your doctor – you can obtain all the vitamins and minerals you need by eating a healthy diet and taking a daily multivitamin supplement.

EXPLAINING THE SYMBOLS

SOLUBLE FIBRE

 HIGH

 MEDIUM

LOW

UNSATURATED FAT

 HIGH

 MEDIUM

LOW

PROTEIN

 HIGH

 MEDIUM

 LOW

CHOLESTEROL

 HIGH

 MEDIUM

 LOW

ANTIOXIDANT

 HIGH

 MEDIUM

 LOW

GLYCAEMIC INDEX

 HIGH

 MEDIUM

 LOW

SATURATED FAT

 HIGH

 MEDIUM

 LOW

INSOLUBLE FIBRE

 HIGH

 MEDIUM

 LOW

HEALTHY EATING PYRAMID

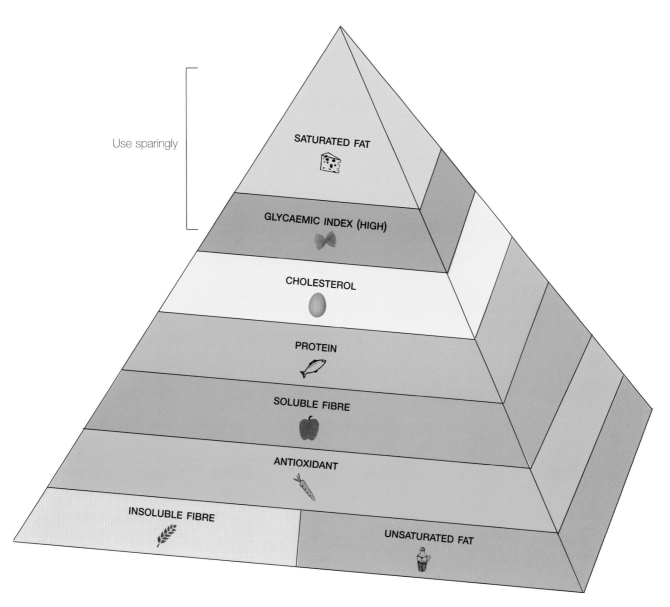

Use sparingly

SATURATED FAT

GLYCAEMIC INDEX (HIGH)

CHOLESTEROL

PROTEIN

SOLUBLE FIBRE

ANTIOXIDANT

INSOLUBLE FIBRE

UNSATURATED FAT

 Saturated Fat: Red meat, goose, duck, cheese, butter, cream, full-fat yoghurt

 Glycaemic Index (HIGH): Rice, white bread, potatoes, desserts, broad beans, prunes, watermelon and pasta

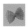 **Cholesterol:** Eggs, butter, cream, cheese, shellfish, pork, lamb, beef (0–1 times daily)

 Protein: Fish, shellfish, free-range chicken, rabbit, wild game, low-fat dairy (1–2 times daily)

 Soluble Fibre: Oats, barley, peas, beans, fruits (e.g. apples, oranges, bananas, walnuts), nuts (2–3 times daily)

 Antioxidant: Spinach, broccoli, garlic, onions, red and orange vegetables and fruit, berries (at most meals)

 Insoluble Fibre: Wheat bran, wholewheat flour, wild rice, grains, cabbage, cauliflower, fruit skins (at most meals)

 Unsaturated Fat: Olive oil, soya beans, avocado, peanuts, salmon, mackerel, tuna, sardines (1–2 times daily)

STRIKING A BALANCE

It is easy to decide which foods you should eat, but more difficult to decide how often to eat them. It is also hard to strike a nutritional balance between foods so that you obtain all the nutrients that your body demands in the correct quantities, yet protect your heart and arteries at the same time. And you will have noticed already from the tables in this book that certain foods are 'good' in the sense that they contain substantial quantities of a desirable ingredient, but 'not so good' in that they contain less desirable ingredients. So how do you do it?

The healthy eating pyramid shown on the previous page indicates how often you should eat the different food groups. For instance, while foods such as cheese and other dairy products are important as part of a balanced diet, you should try to use these sparingly because of the high levels of saturated fat they contain.

It combines sound nutritional advice with common sense. Use it to plan your diet, both for control of your diabetes (or pre-diabetes) and for general good health.

HOW TO COOK HEALTHILY

There is little point in choosing healthy heart ingredients and recipes if you cook them in a way that is in itself unhealthy. For diabetics in particular it is important to choose cooking methods that not only help reduce cholesterol and saturated fats, so reducing the risk of heart disease and keeping the calorie count low, but maximize the nutritional value of each dish. These techniques are effective, but may require a little practice:

- Baking – good for vegetables, fruit, poultry and lean meat, as well as for puddings; you may need a little extra liquid

- Braising or stewing – brown first, on top of the stove, then cook in a small quantity of liquid; if you leave the dish in a refrigerator you can remove the chilled fat and then reheat it

- Grilling – on a rack, so that fat can drain away

- Microwaving – place the food between two paper towels to drain fat away while it cooks

- Poaching – in a covered pan of the correct size, so that you use the minimum liquid

- Roasting – on a rack so that the food does not sit in fat; baste with fat-free liquids, such as wine or lemon juice

- Sautéing – use a high heat and a small amount of non-stick cooking spray, or just cook without spray if you have a good-quality non-stick pan

- Steaming – in a perforated basket over simmering water; add seasoning to the water for extra flavour

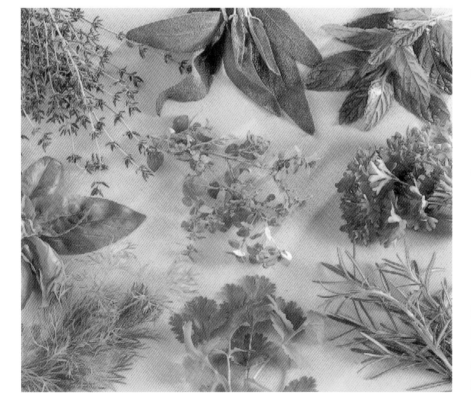

Use chopped, fresh herbs to flavour your sauces rather than salt. The best way to appreciate herbs is when they are freshly picked.

- Stir-frying – in a wok, using a small amount of non-stick cooking spray or a tiny amount of olive oil.

You can also increase flavour, reduce fat and salt content, and make the most of your ingredients' nutritional value if you

REMEMBER TO:

- Check labels for common ingredients, such as soy sauce, baking soda and monosodium glutamate – these all contain high levels of sodium and should be used very sparingly, if at all

- Make your own stock rather than using pre-prepared cubes, which can be high in salt

- Steam vegetables, for preference, in order to maximize both their flavour and nutritional value

  - Cook lightly to preserve vitamin content (but cook meats and other foods that may harbour disease-producing organisms thoroughly)

  - Choose extra virgin olive oil and vinegar rather than salted, pre-prepared salad dressings

  - Wash canned vegetables before use – by doing so you can substantially reduce their salt content

  - Use only one egg yolk when making scrambled eggs or omelettes, but mix in two or three extra egg whites

  - Trim as much fat as you can from meat before you cook it and remove the skin from poultry

  - Choose lean, low-fat meats, such as game (but, again, remember to remove the skin) and venison

  - Drain oil from canned fish and rinse the fish in water before you use it

  - Use herbs, lemon juice, wine, and freshly ground pepper to enhance flavours.

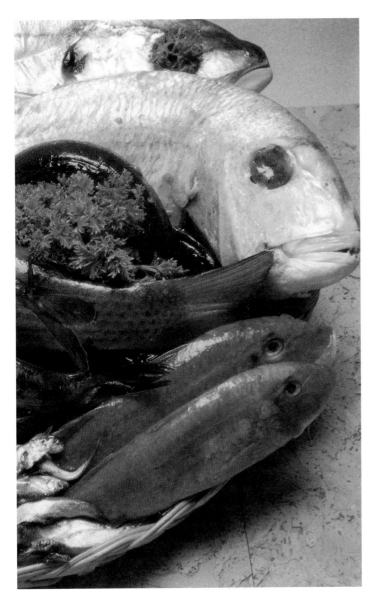

Salt-water fish are a superior source of nutrients, which are vital to growth and good health. Fish yield high amounts of proteins, vitamins, minerals and unsaturated fats.

FISH STOCK

Ingredients

1 kg fish bones, heads (with gills removed) and tails
  (sole or plaice are tastiest, but any other white, non-
  only fish will do)
1 large onion, coarsely chopped
2 shallots, coarsely chopped
2 ribs of celery, tops included, coarsely chopped
2 large carrots, scrubbed but not peeled, coarsely
  chopped
2 bay leaves
2 cloves
6 sprigs of parsley, coarsely chopped
1 tbsp peppercorns
Lemon rind from half a lemon
Cold water to cover

Method

Place everything in a stockpot and bring to simmering
point – do not allow to boil. Simmer for 20–30
minutes, but no longer or the stock will become bitter.
Strain through cheesecloth or use a non-metallic
colander. Reduce the strained stock by boiling, if
required. Use or freeze as required.

VEGETABLE STOCK

Ingredients

3 large carrots, scrubbed but not peeled, coarsely
  chopped
1 turnip, coarsely chopped
2 onions, coarsely chopped
2 leeks, coarsely chopped
4 ribs of celery, including tops, coarsely chopped
coarsely chopped trimmings from cauliflower, spinach,
  broccoli or any other vegetables, so long as they are
  fresh and clean. Always use fresh vegetables.
1 cup any dried beans, having been soaked overnight, if
  necessary; or use rice or barley
2 tbsp olive oil
1 bouquet garni, which includes 3 sprigs parsley,
  1 sprig thyme and 1 bay leaf
1 tbsp peppercorns
Approx 3 litres of cold water for 1 kg vegetables

Method

Warm the olive oil in a stockpot, add the vegetables
and simmer, stirring continuously for 15 minutes until
they start to colour slightly. Then add the water and
the other ingredients and bring to simmering point.
Simmer for at least 2 hours, adding more water if
necessary. Then strain through cheesecloth or use a
non-metallic colander. Use or freeze, as required.

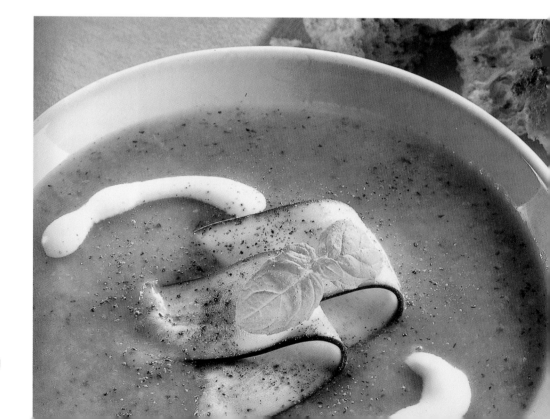

*Use the stocks for the
basis of soups and
stews.*

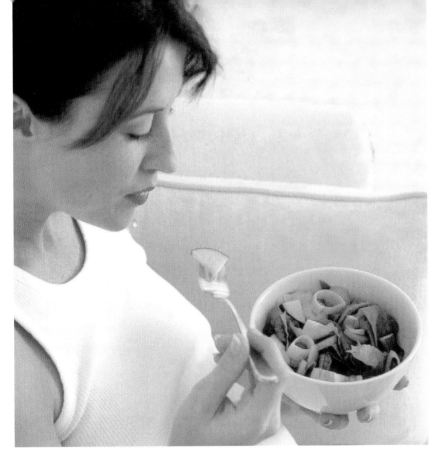

Eating nutritiously is important, as well as getting plenty of exercise. If you need a snack, then the best things to eat are fresh fruit and vegetables that are high in vitamins and minerals.

THE HEALTHY LIFESTYLE

Eating diabetic- and heart-friendly dishes is only one part of a healthy lifestyle. It is especially important that diabetics reduce blood glucose levels and blood pressure, lower their cholesterol levels and promote cardiovascular health. In order to do this you should also:

Give up smoking – if you smoke, you are at more than double the risk of having a heart attack than a non-smoker, and you are considerably more likely not to survive a heart attack

Manage stress – use relaxation techniques and anger-management methods to cope with stress and keep your blood pressure low

Lose weight – if you are overweight, you are between two and six times more likely to develop insulin resistance, high blood pressure and diabetes; but resist the temptation to go on a crash diet, because permanent weight loss is only achieved by reducing your calorific input and increasing the amount of exercise you do in the long term: aim to lose approximately between half a kg and three quarter kg (1 lb and 1.5 lb) a week

Cut down on alcohol – there's evidence to suggest that two units of alcohol, and especially of red wine, can reduce blood pressure, but more than this can increase blood pressure; it can also make hypoglycaemia more severe, while masking awareness of the problem

Lead an active life – even small amounts of physical activity, for example walking or gardening, can reduce the risk of developing diabetes and heart disease.

CHICKEN STOCK

Ingredients:
The bones of a chicken, and, if available, a ham bone
  or a veal knuckle (ask your butcher for one)
2 leeks, coarsely chopped
2 large carrots, scrubbed but not peeled, coarsely
  chopped
3 large onions, coarsely chopped
2 ribs of celery, tops included, coarsely chopped
6 sprigs of parsley, coarsely chopped
1 large clove of garlic
2 cloves
1 tbsp peppercorns
Lemon rind from half a lemon

Method:
Place the bones in a stockpot and cover with cold water. Bring to simmering point – do not allow to boil. Simmer for at least an hour, then add all other ingredients and more cold water to cover, if necessary. Return to simmering point and simmer for another 2 hours. Then strain through cheesecloth or use a non-metallic colander. Refrigerate, and when stock has set remove any fat from the top. Use or freeze, as required.

TABLES

These tables give the nutritional values for the main ingredients used in the recipes that follow. To eat healthily and minimize your risk of developing diabetes, to control your insulin levels if you have the condition, and also to minimize the risk of developing heart disease and other complications of diabetes, the major part of your diet should consist of foods with a low or medium glycaemic index, a low fat content, moderate protein levels and a high fibre content. Use the Healthy Eating Pyramid on page 21 as a guide to proportions.

Remember that carrying excess weight is a major risk for developing heart problems, and watch your calorie intake, too. Doctors recommend that men with a sedentary lifestyle – that of an office worker, say – should eat 2,700 calories a day, while women should eat 2,000. In order to lose weight gradually, at the rate of half kg (1 lb) a week, you need to reduce this figure by 500 calories.

Food	Quantity	Glycaemic index	Fat	Protein	Fibre	Calories
Meat and Dairy						
Cheese, feta	20 g	6	M	4	0	80
Cheese, reduced fat	20 g	4.5	M	7	0	70
Chicken skinless	100 g	5	L	30	0	150
Crème fraîche, low fat	100 ml	17.5	M	3	0	800
Egg	1 medium	5.5	M	6	0	80
Lean beef, lamb, pork	100 g	7	M	30	0	190
Milk, low fat	250 ml	2.5	L	8	0	102
Rabbit	100 g	4.5	L	30	0	160
Wild fowl	100 g	6	L	30	0	155
Yogurt	100 ml	0	L	5	0	40
Fish						
Herring, salmon	100 g	11	L	20	0	180
Mackerel	100 g	18	L	25	0	220
Sardine	100 g	2	L	15	0	65
Shellfish	100 g	1	L	15	0	105
Trout	100 g	6	L	20	0	155
Tuna	100 g	3	L	20	0	120
White fish	100 g	2	L	20	0	90

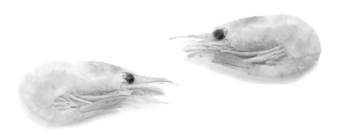

Prawns are an excellent low-calorie food choice, and they are a rich source of protein, vitamins and minerals.

Food	Quantity	Glycaemic index	Fat	Protein	Fibre	Calories
Fruit						
Apple	1 medium	0	L	0.5	2	45
Apricot	3	0	M	1.5	2	30
Banana	1 small	0.5	M	1	1	90
Berries, fresh	100 g	0	L	0.5	1	30
Dried fruit	50 g	0	M	0.5	4	80
Grapefruit	half	0	L	0.5	1	30
Melon	slice	0	M	0.5	1	50
Nectarine, peach	1 medium	0	L	0.5	1	35
Orange	1 medium	0	L	1.5	3	50

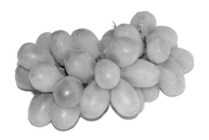

Fruit is easily digested, is an excellent source of fibre and has a moderate glycaemic index value.

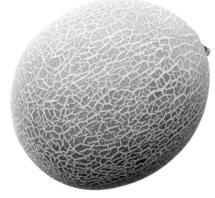

Food	Quantity	Glycaemic index	Fat	Protein	Fibre	Calories
Vegetables						
Eggplant	100 g	0	L	0.5	2	75
Avocado	½ medium	15	L	2	3.5	150
Beans	100 g	0.5	L	6	4	100
Beetroot	small	0	L	0.5	0.5	25
Broccoli	100 g	0	L	1.5	2.5	25
Cabbage	50 g	0	L	1	1	7
Carrot	50 g	0	L	0.5	1	12

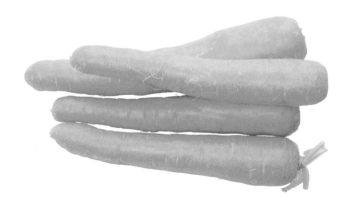

Carrots contain beta-carotene (providing vitamin A value) and cooking carrots actually enhances the digestibility of the beta-carotene.

Food	Quantity	Glycaemic index	Fat	Protein	Fibre	Calories
Vegetables (*continued*)						
Cauliflower	50 g	0	L	1	1.5	20
Green beans	100 g	0	L	1.5	2.5	20
Onions	medium	0	L	1	1.4	30
Peas	100 g	0	L	3.5	6	60
Peppers	100 g	0	L	1	2.5	30
Potatoes, new	3	0	M	1.5	3	100
Soyabean	100 g	7	L	8	6	120
Spinach	50 g cooked	0	L	1	1	10
Squash, butternut	100 g	0	M	1	1.5	30
Sweetcorn	100 g	0. 5	M	2.5	1.5	95
Tofu	100 g	4	L	8	0	70
Tomato	medium	0	L	1	1	15

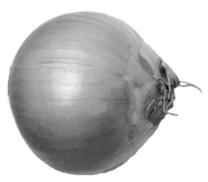

Eating raw onions can help to reduce cholesterol levels because they increase levels of high-density lipoproteins. As a result, they can help lower blood pressure and so reduce the risk of heart disease or a stroke.

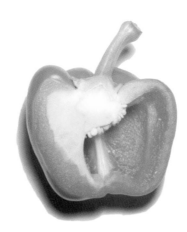

Peppers are low in calories and are especially rich in vitamins A and C. Surprisingly, a pepper contains three to four times more vitamin C than an orange. They do not contain any fat and help to stimulate the circulation.

Food	Quantity	Glycaemic index	Fat	Protein	Fibre	Calories
Cereal, Nuts, Pulses						
Barley	50 g raw	1	L	2	1	140
Chickpeas	100 g	3	L	5	4	110
Lentils	100 g	0.5	L	8	2	100
Oats	50 g raw	1	L	4	3	140
Pasta, wholegrain	100 g	1	L	5	4	120
Rice, brown, basmati	100 g	0	M	3.5	1	200
Walnuts	2 tbsp	8	L	2	1	80
Wild rice	100 g	0	M	3	1	100

BREAKFASTS

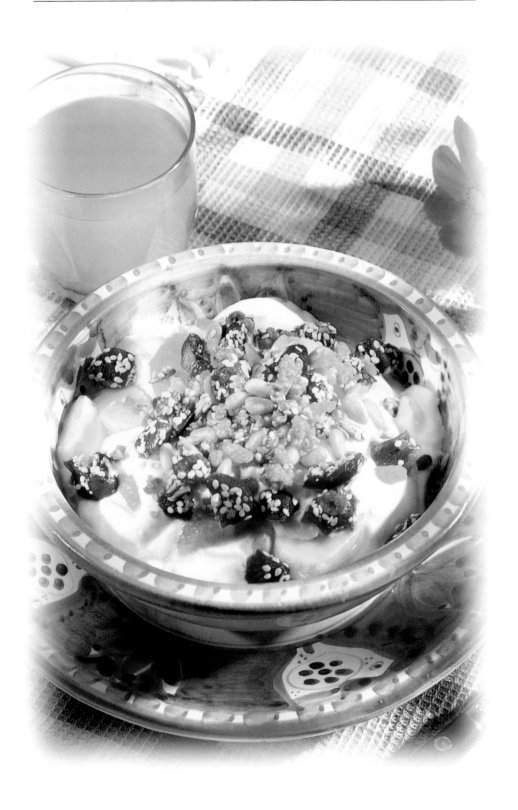

HOMEMADE MUESLI

MAKES ABOUT **255 g**

*Many whole-food stores sell bags of mixed grains ready for making muesli.
Otherwise, keep the mixture as plain or as varied as you like – a simple combination
of oatmeal (an excellent source of soluble fibre) and fruit is perfectly good.*

167 g oatmeal

125 g bran

62.5 g wheat or millet flakes

75 g raisins

75 g golden raisins

112.5 g chopped dried apple rings

150 g chopped ready-to-eat dried
   apricots

150 g chopped walnuts

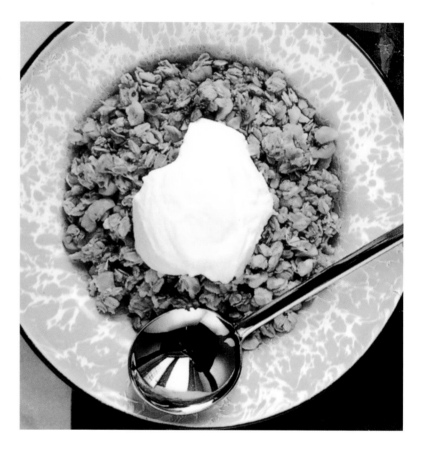

1 Mix all the ingredients in a large bowl, then store
the muesli in an airtight container in a cool, dry
place.

2 Serve with milk (skimmed or low fat) or natural
yoghurt. Fresh fruit, such as banana, grapes or
peach, may be served with the muesli. For a
special breakfast, combine a selection of chopped
fresh fruits with the muesli.

NUTRITIONAL VALUES

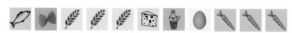

GRAPEFRUIT, MELON AND GRAPE COCKTAILS

SERVES **4**

Like other citrus fruits, grapefruit is believed to slow down the rate of sugar metabolism. Here the fruit is transformed into three lively cocktails to start the day or begin a meal.

GRAPEFRUIT COCKTAIL

2 large juicy grapefruit

1 Peel the grapefruit and remove all the pith. Hold the fruit over a bowl and use a sharp serrated knife to cut in towards the middle of the fruit, removing the fleshy segments and leaving behind the membranes that seperate them.

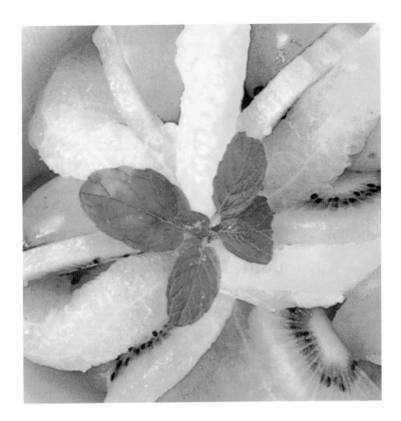

MELON COCKTAIL

5 cm piece fresh ginger root, peeled and
    chopped

a little water

1 tbsp artificial sweetner

1 tbsp rose-water

¹/₂ honeydew melon

large wedge watermelon

1 Place the ginger in a small saucepan with water to cover. Bring to the boil, cover and simmer for 30 minutes, making sure the water does not evaporate. At the end of cooking boil the ginger, if necessary, until the liquid is reduced to 2 tablespoons or slightly less. Leave to cool, then stir in the artificial sweetner and rose-water.

2 Discard the seeds and peel from both types of melon, then cut them into small, neat cubes. Mix the melon with the grapefruit and strain the ginger juice over. Chill for at least 30 minutes before serving.

GRAPE COCKTAIL

125 g seedless green grapes

2 kiwi fruit, peeled, halved and sliced

4 mint sprigs

1 Leave small grapes whole and halve larger ones, then mix them with the grapefruit. Add the kiwi fruit and mint, then mix lightly.

NUTRITIONAL VALUES

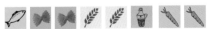

RED DEVIL JUICE

SERVES **4**

A healthy and refreshing juice drink for breakfast with an added kick to it!

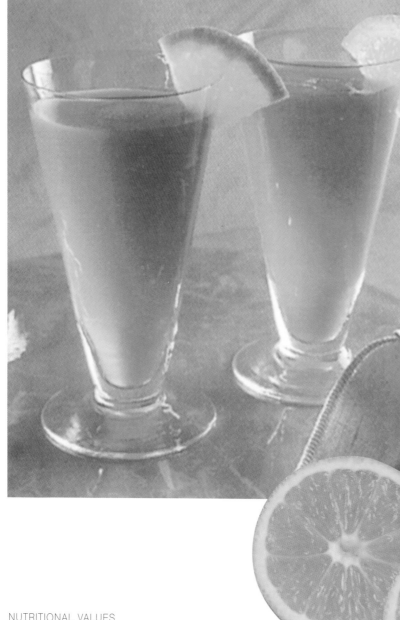

900 ml tomato juice

3–4 drops Tabasco

150 ml orange juice, freshly
  squeezed

TO GARNISH

ice cubes

4 orange rind twists

4 small celery sticks

1 Mix the tomato juice and
tabasco together. Add the
orange juice and stir well to
blend.

2 Pour into 4 small tumblers.
Add ice cubes, garnish with
orange twists and place a
celery stick in each glass.
Serve immediately.

NUTRITIONAL VALUES

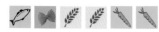

HERB BREAKFAST OMELETTE

SERVES **4**

A quick and easy cheese and egg recipe mixed with herbs that is full of protein to help start the day.

4 eggs, lightly beaten

56 g cottage cheese

1 tbsp parsley, finely chopped

2 tsp fresh thyme, finely chopped

14 g unsalted butter

2 tomatoes, chopped

150 g chopped ready-to-eat dried
   apricots

150 g chopped walnuts

TO SERVE

wholemeal toast

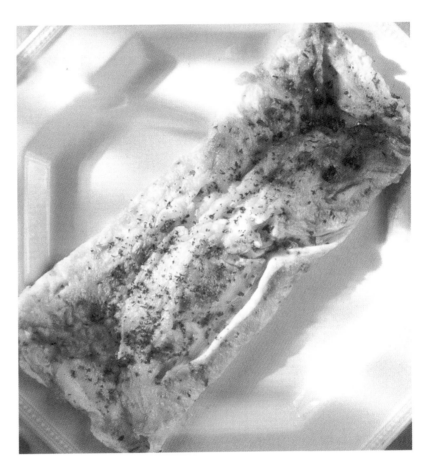

1 Place the eggs, cheese, herbs and Worcestershire sauce in a bowl and whisk together.

2 Place the unsalted butter in a non-stick omelette pan and place over a medium heat to melt.

3 Pour in the egg mix and draw the edge of the omelette to the centre of the pan as it becomes firm. Tip the pan gently to allow the uncooked egg mixture to flow to the sides of the pan.

4 When it is lightly set, sprinkle with the tomato and cook gently for 1 minute.

5 Fold in half and transfer to a warmed serving plate.

6 Cut into 4 portions and serve immediately with wholemeal toast, if wished.

NUTRITIONAL VALUES

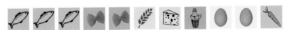

BREAKFAST CRUNCH

SERVES **4 – 6**

A delicious breakfast in a bowl, packed with lots of fruity goodness!

30 g sunflower seeds

30 g pine kernels

30 g sesame seeds

2 oranges

75 g dried figs, chopped

2 large bananas

600 ml Greek yoghurt

NUTRITIONAL VALUES

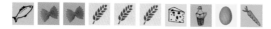

1 Using a dry frying pan, roast the sunflower seeds and pine kernels for 3 minutes over medium heat, then add the sesame seeds and roast for a further 3 minutes, stirring to give even browning. Remove the pan from the heat.

2 Coarsely grate the peel from 1 orange and add to the pan with the dried figs. Stir until well combined and cook for 2 minutes. Leave to cool.

3 Remove the peel and pith from the oranges and cut them into pieces. Slice the bananas and mix with the oranges and yoghurt, divide among 4 dishes and top each with the fig and seeds mixture. Serve at once.

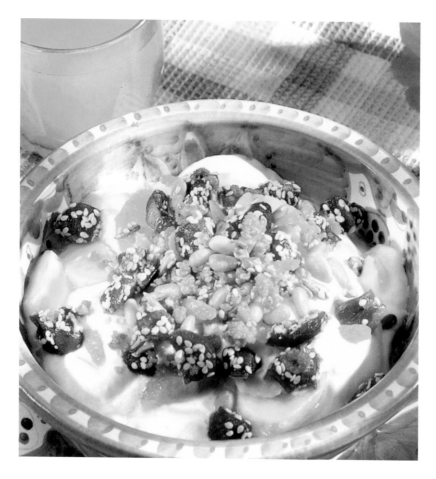

APPLE DROP BISCUITS

SERVES **4**

This healthy version of a breakfast favourite is filled with chunks of crisp apple which are complemented by the cinnamon-spiced yoghurt sauce.

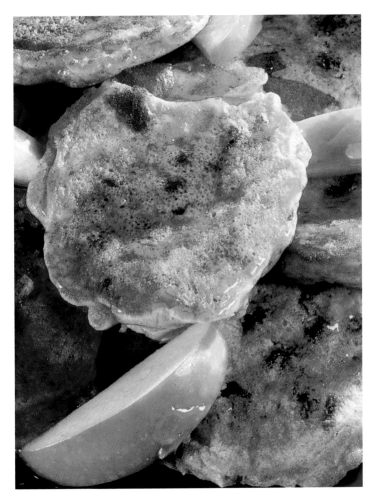

80 ml skimmed milk

1 green dessert apple, cored and chopped

1 tbsp raisins

vegetable oil

FOR THE BISCUITS

60 g wholewheat flour

1 tsp baking powder

1 tsp caster sugar

1 medium egg, beaten

FOR THE YOGHURT SAUCE

170 g low-fat plain yoghurt

$1/_2$ tsp ground cinnamon

1 tsp honey

1 Sift the flour and baking powder for the biscuits into a mixing bowl and stir in the sugar. Make a well in the centre and beat in the egg and milk to make a smooth batter. Stir in the apple and raisins, mixing well.

2 Brush a heavy pan with a little oil and warm over medium heat. Divide the batter into 8 equal portions and drop 4 portions into the pan, spacing them well apart.

3 Cook for 2–3 minutes until the top of each drop biscuit begins to bubble. Turn the biscuits over and cook for 1 minute. Transfer to a warmed plate while cooking the remaining 4 biscuits.

4 Mix the yoghurt sauce ingredients together in a bowl. Serve with the hot drop biscuits.

NUTRITIONAL VALUES

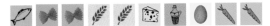

BANANA COCKTAIL

SERVES **4**

This is a nourishing 'spoon drink' to serve to people caught up in the morning rush. The honey and citrus fruits compensate for any loss of dairy flavour as a result of using skimmed milk.

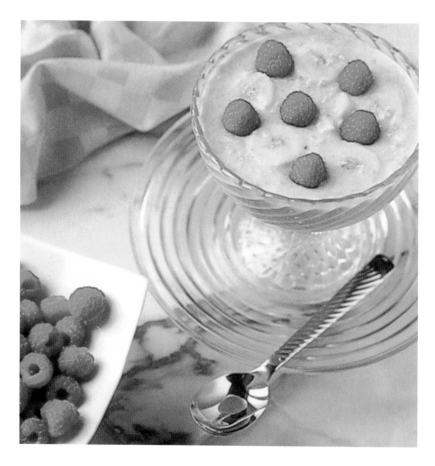

100 g rolled porridge oats

200 ml skimmed milk

4 tbsp clear honey

2 large dessert apples, peeled, cored and grated

2 medium bananas, thinly sliced

juice of 1 lemon

juice of 1 orange

2 tsp grated orange rind

300 ml plain low-fat yoghurt

GARNISH

4 tsp dark muscovado sugar

2 tbsp fresh or frozen berries, or orange segments

1 Soak the porridge oats in skimmed milk overnight.

2 In the morning stir in all the remaining ingredients and divide the mixture among 4 individual serving glasses, such as sundae glasses.

3 Decorate each glass with whatever fruit is available. Oatcakes make a very good accompaniment.

NUTRITIONAL VALUES

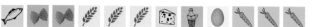

LIGHT MEALS

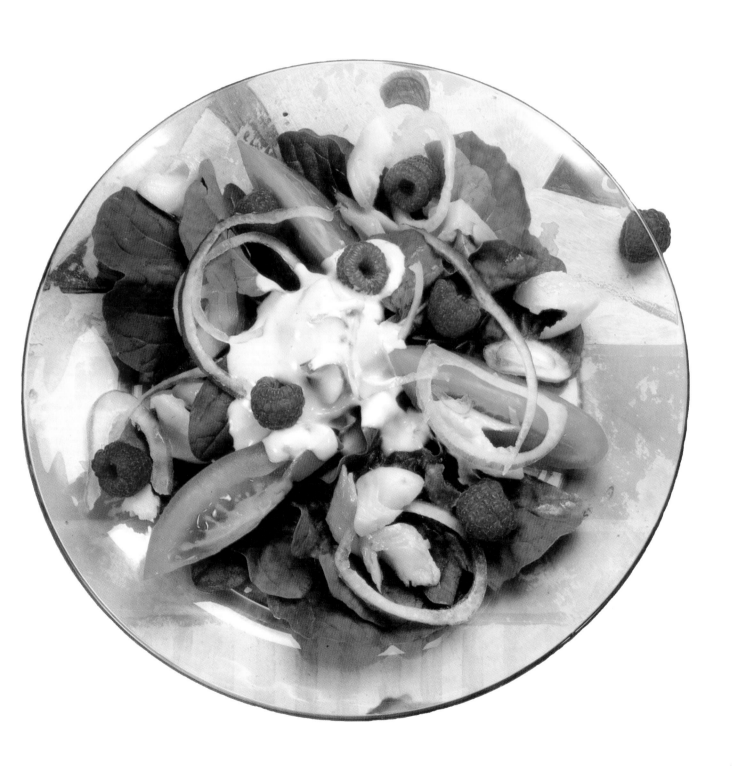

GARLIC NEW POTATOES

SERVES **4**

New potatoes are just young potatoes of any variety. Choose firm, well-shaped and blemish-free potatoes of roughly equal size, so that they all cook in the same amount of time.

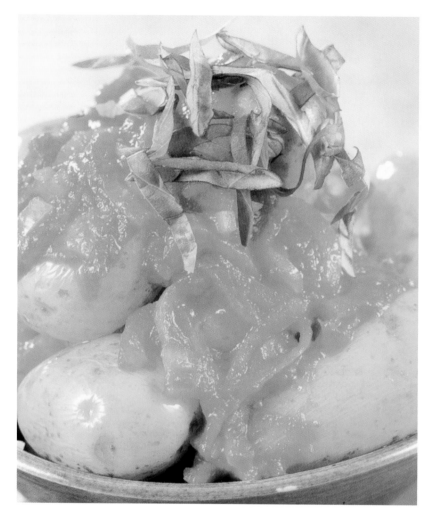

450 g new potatoes, lightly
    scrubbed

2 tbsp olive oil

2 garlic cloves, peeled and crushed

1 tbsp fresh basil, chopped

FOR THE SAUCE

1 small onion, quartered and thinly
    sliced

1 tsp paprika

pinch of cayenne pepper

1 tsp fennel seed

300 ml passata

300 ml vegetable stock

2 tbsp fresh basil, chopped

fresh basil, to garnish

1   Line a steamer tier with foil, making an edge to form a dish. Put the potatoes, oil, garlic and basil in the foil.

2   Place the sauce ingredients in the base of the steamer and bring to the boil. Cook the potatoes, covered, over the sauce for 45 minutes until the potatoes are tender. Garnish with basil, and serve with the sauce.

NUTRITIONAL VALUES

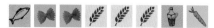

SALAD NIÇOISE

SERVES **4**

This makes a delicious lunch, appetizer for a dinner party or buffet salad, with crusty wholegrain bread.

450 g potatoes, boiled

250 g green beans, fresh or frozen

200 g can tuna fish

150 ml vinaigrette

4 tomatoes, skinned and sliced

¼ cucumber

1 hard-boiled egg

12 black or green olives, stones removed

6 anchovy fillets, cut into thin slices

TO GARNISH

small cherry tomatoes

NUTRITIONAL VALUES

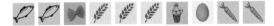

1 Cook the potatoes in their skins until tender. Remove the skins and dice finely. Cook the beans in a small amount of boiling water for about 6 minutes. Frozen beans can be used; cook as directed on the packet.

2 Mix the potatoes, beans and half the tuna fish with three-quarters of the vinaigrette.

3 Arrange the sliced tomatoes on the bottom and around the bowl, arrange thinly sliced cucumber on top, and sprinkle with a little vinaigrette. Place a few chunks of tuna fish on the tomato and cucumber.

4 The egg may be cut into slices or wedges and can be used on top as a garnish or arranged to make a bed for the beans, potatoes and tuna fish mixture.

5 Arrange the fish mixture in the middle and arrange the anchovies in a diamond-shaped pattern on the beans, decorating each space with an olive. Pour over any remaining dressing.

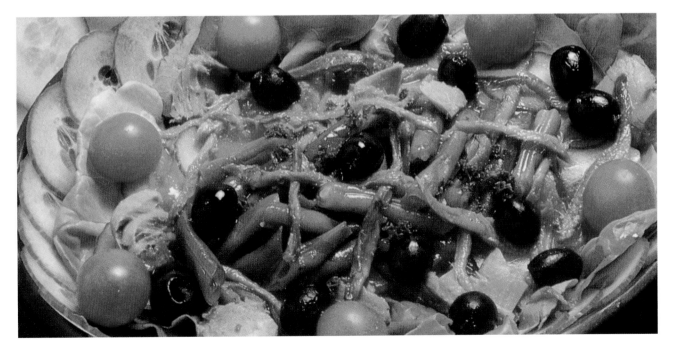

PEPPER AND TOMATO BRUSCHETTA

SERVES **4 – 6**

Serve this bright red mixture of roasted tomatoes and peppers on crisply toasted bread that has been rubbed with a clove of garlic. This Italian hors d'oeuvre can be followed by a main course of grilled sardines, roasted chicken or pasta.

4 small to medium-sized
 tomatoes

pepper to taste

2 tbsp extra virgin olive oil

4 red peppers, roasted, peeled
 and diced

2–3 garlic cloves, chopped

few drops of white wine vinegar
 or balsamic vinegar, to taste

few fresh basil leaves, torn, or
 other sweet Mediterranean
 herb such as oregano or
 marjoram

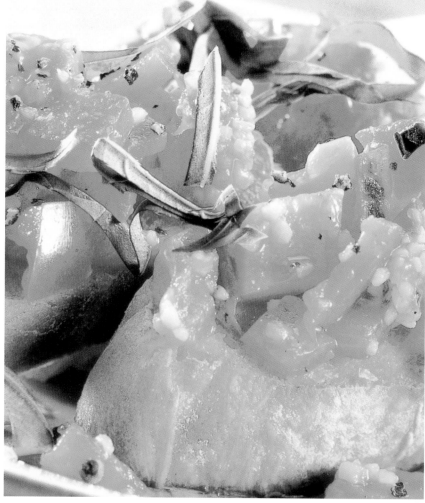

1 Cut the tomatoes into half and sprinkle the cut half lightly with pepper.

2 Heat a tablespoon of the olive oil in a heavy frying pan just large enough to take all the tomato halves. When the frying pan is hot, place the tomatoes skin-side down and cook for a few minutes over high heat until the tomatoes are charred underneath, then turn them carefully, reduce the heat to about medium-high, and cook, covered, until done. Do not overcook.

3 Remove from the heat and leave, covered, until cool.

4 Dice the roasted tomatoes and combine them, with their juices, with the diced peppers and garlic. Season with pepper, and add the vinegar and remaining olive oil. Serve at room temperature, sprinkled with the herbs.

NUTRITIONAL VALUES

YELLOW PEPPERS & SUN DRIED TOMATOES

SERVES **4**

Homemade sun-dried tomatoes are best with this – they are tender and more flavoursome than the bottled variety, which can be tough. This appetizer is delicious on small pieces of French bread or crisp crostini-like toasts.

3 yellow peppers, cut into bite-sized pieces

4–5 tbsp extra-virgin olive oil

4–5 cloves garlic, chopped

400 g ripe tomatoes, diced (or 400 g can chopped tomatoes)

freshly ground black pepper

8–10 marinated sun-dried tomatoes, cut into quarters

1 tbsp balsamic vinegar or to taste

2–3 tsp capers, rinsed and drained

fresh chopped parsley, to garnish

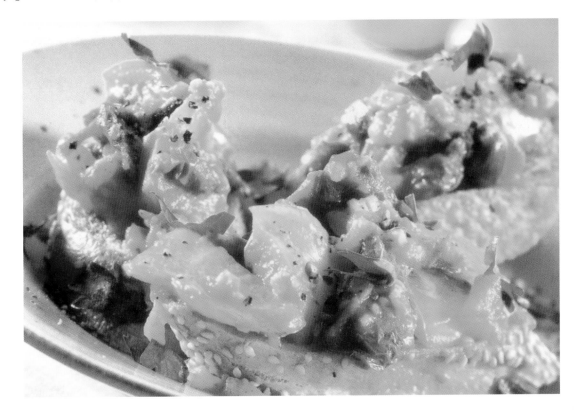

1 Brown the peppers in the olive oil for about 7 minutes, long enough to lightly brown them without them turning too soft.

2 Add half the garlic, the diced tomatoes and pepper, and cook over high heat until the tomatoes reduce to a thick paste.

3 Stir in the sun-dried tomatoes, balsamic vinegar, capers, and remaining garlic, and cool to room temperature to serve. Garnish with fresh parsley if liked.

NUTRITIONAL VALUES

PASTA WITH WALDORF SALAD

SERVES **4**

This recipe is based on the famous Waldorf salad, and every serious cook has their own interpretation. Try this salad as it gives an exciting new twist to the original recipe.

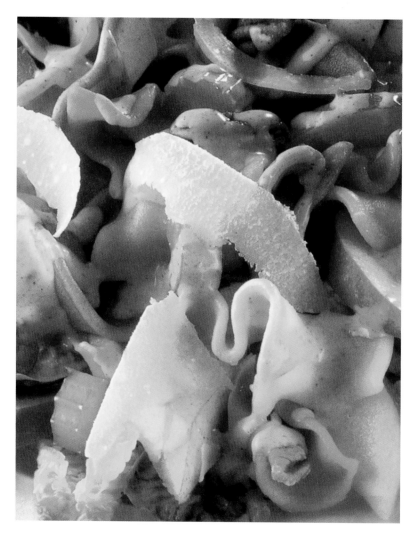

2 red apples, rinsed, cored and thinly sliced

2 ripe pears, peeled, cored and sliced

juice of 1 lemon

4 celery stalks, trimmed and sliced

65 g pecan halves

225 g fresh pasta, such as tri-coloured brandelle

1 small head romaine lettuce

freshly shaved Romano cheese

FOR THE DRESSING

3 tbsp reduced calorie mayonnaise

2 tbsp yoghurt

1–2 tsp medium hot curry powder

1 Place the apples and pears in a bowl, pour over the lemon juice, and toss lightly.

2 Add the sliced celery and pecan halves, and mix lightly.

3 Cook the pasta in plenty of boiling water for 1–2 minutes or until firm to the bite. Drain and add to the celery.

4 Blend together the reduced calorie mayonnaise, yoghurt and curry powder to taste, reserve. Rinse the lettuce and use to line a salad bowl. Pile the prepared salad into the centre and drizzle over the dressing. Sprinkle with the freshly shaved Romano cheese.

NUTRITIONAL VALUES

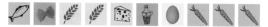

VEGETABLE JAMBALAYA

SERVES **4**

This is a classic Caribbean dish, usually made with spicy sausage, but this vegetarian version packs just as much of a punch and tastes wonderful.

generous 30 g long grain rice

30 g wild rice

1 aubergine, sliced and quartered

1 tsp salt substitute
  (see page 15)

1 onion, chopped

1 celery stalk, trimmed and sliced

198 ml vegetable broth

2 garlic cloves, minced

100 g baby corn

100 g green beans, trimmed

100 g baby carrots

100 g canned chopped tomatoes

4 tsp tomato purée

1 tsp creole seasoning

1 tsp chilli sauce

chopped fresh parsley, to garnish

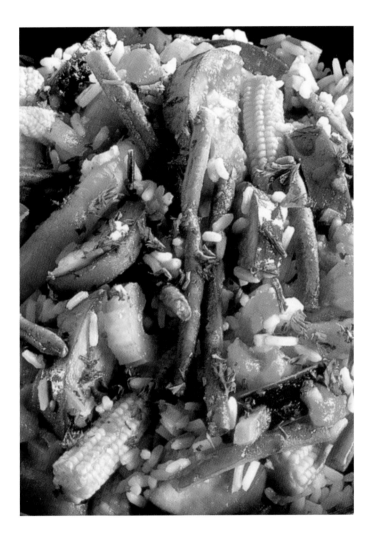

1 Cook the rices in boiling water for 20 minutes or until cooked. Drain well.

2 Meanwhile, place the aubergine pieces in a colander, sprinkle with salt substitute, and leave to stand for 20 minutes. Wash and pat dry with paper towels.

3 Put the aubergine, onion, celery and broth in a non-stick pan and cook for 5 minutes, stirring.

4 Add the garlic, corn, beans, carrots, tomatoes, tomato purée, creole seasoning and chilli sauce. Bring the mixture to the boil, reduce the heat and cook for 20 minutes more until the vegetables are just cooked.

5 Stir in the drained rice and cook for 5 minutes more. Garnish with parsley and serve.

NUTRITIONAL VALUES

SAUTÉED FLAGEOLET BEANS WITH FUSILLI

SERVES **2-4**

A garlicky dish, made with fresh tarragon to enhance the delicate flavours. Serve as a main course or as an accompaniment.

275 g dried fusilli (short twists)

dash of olive oil, plus 4 tbsp

3 garlic cloves, crushed

1 large onion, sliced

2 tbsp chopped fresh tarragon

400 g can flageolet beans, drained

salt substitute (see page 15) and freshly ground
   black pepper

NUTRITIONAL VALUES

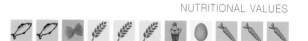

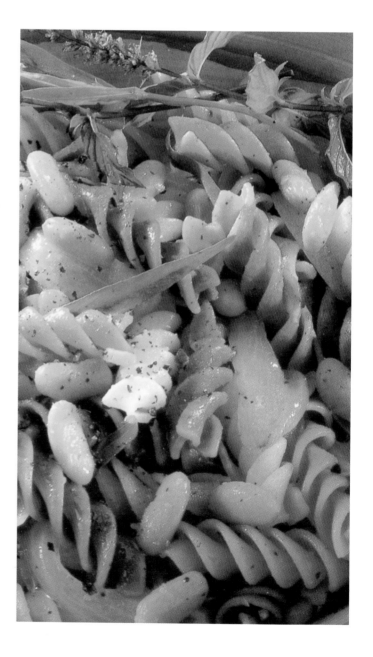

1   Bring a large saucepan of water to the boil and
    add the fusilli with a dash of olive oil.

2   Cook for about 10 minutes, stirring
    occasionally, until tender. Drain and set aside.

3   Heat the olive oil in a frying pan and sauté the
    garlic and onion for about 5 minutes, until the
    onion has browned slightly.

4   Add the tarragon and beans and season with
    the salt substitute and freshly ground black
    pepper. Cook for 2–3 minutes, then stir in the
    fusilli.

5   Cook for a further 3–5 minutes, to heat
    through. Serve with a crisp green salad.

PIMENTO PASTA

A quick store-cupboard recipe for a last-minute supper surprise.

1 Bring a large saucepan of water to the boil and add the spaghetti with a dash of olive oil. Cook for about 10 minutes, stirring occasionally, until tender.

2 Drain and return to the saucepan. Set aside, covered, to keep warm.

3 Heat the remaining olive oil in a frying pan and add the garlic and sliced pimento. Stir-fry for 3–5 minutes, then tip into the warm spaghetti. Stir to combine.

4 Serve with a little freshly shredded Parmesan cheese, if desired.

350 g dried spaghetti

dash of olive oil, plus 2 tbsp

2 garlic cloves, crushed

400 g can red pimento, thinly sliced

salt substitute (see page 15) and freshly ground black pepper

freshly shredded Parmesan cheese, to serve (optional)

NUTRITIONAL VALUES

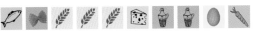

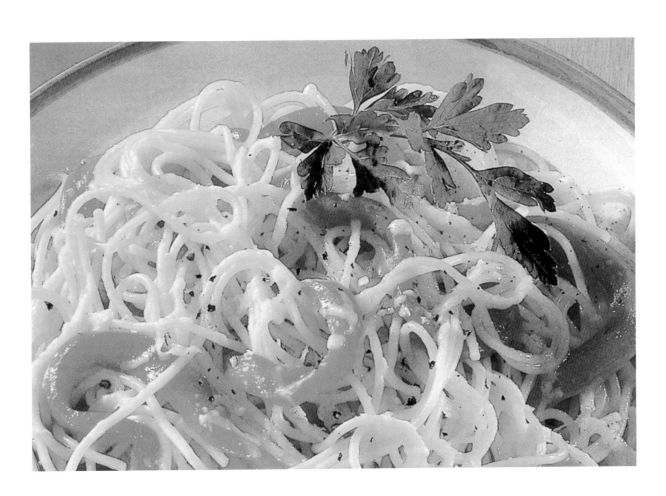

PROVENÇAL GREEN BEANS WITH PASTA

SERVES **4 – 6**

A delicious way to serve green beans, piping hot with freshly grated parmesan cheese.

2 tbsp olive oil

3 garlic cloves, crushed

1 onion, chopped

3 tbsp chopped fresh thyme

450 g haricot beans, topped and tailed

400 g can chopped tomatoes

50 g tomato purée

425 ml vegetable stock

150 ml dry red wine

salt substitute (see page 15) and freshly
  ground black pepper

450 g dried pasta (any shapes)

2 tbsp olive oil

freshly grated parmesan cheese

1 Heat the oil in a large frying pan and sauté the garlic and onion for about 3 minutes, until softened.

2 Add the thyme, beans, tomatoes, tomato purée, vegetable stock and wine, season with salt substitute and freshly ground pepper and stir well to combine. Cover and cook gently for 25–30 minutes, until the beans are tender.

3 Remove the cover and cook for a further 5–8 minutes, stirring occasionally, until the sauce has thickened slightly.

4 Meanwhile, bring a large saucepan of water to the boil and add the pasta with a dash of olive oil. Cook for about 10 minutes, stirring occasionally, until tender.

5 Drain and return to the saucepan. Toss in olive oil and freshly ground pepper. Serve the beans with the hot pasta and freshly grated parmesan cheese.

NUTRITIONAL VALUES

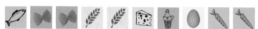

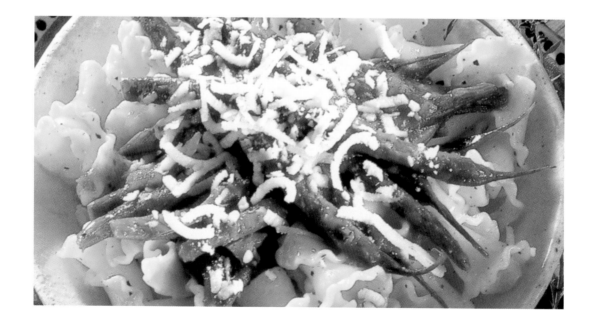

PASTA AL POMODORO

SERVES **4 – 6**

Any pasta shapes would be suitable for this recipe, so use whatever you have in the cupboard. The sauce is quick and simple, making this dish a perfect supper for unexpected guests.

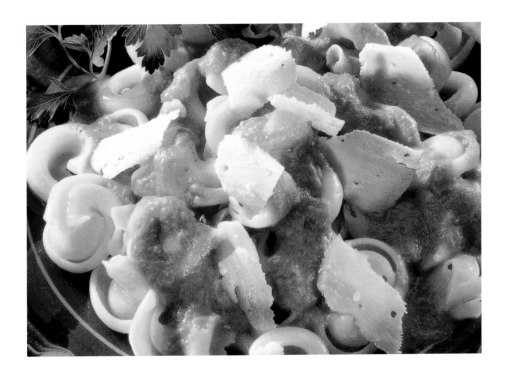

450 g dried pasta

2 tbsp olive oil

2 garlic cloves, crushed

1 onion, chopped

450 g carton sieved tomatoes

salt substitute (see page 15) and freshly
   ground black pepper

fresh flat parsley sprigs, to garnish

slivers of fresh Parmesan cheese, to serve

1 Bring a saucepan of water to the boil and add the pasta with a dash of olive oil. Cook for about 10 minutes, stirring occasionally, until tender.

2 Drain and set aside, covered, to keep warm.

3 In a large frying pan, sauté the garlic and onion in the olive oil for about 3 minutes, until softened. Stir in the tomatoes and season with salt substitute and freshly ground black pepper.

4 Simmer the sauce for about 10 minutes then serve with the pasta, garnished with parsley sprigs and sprinkled with slivers of fresh Parmesan cheese.

NUTRITIONAL VALUES

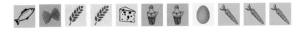

TOMATO AND PASTA SALAD

SERVES **6 – 8**

Orecchiette are small ear-shaped pasta. If they are not available, gnocchi pasta shapes (dumplings) will work just as well.

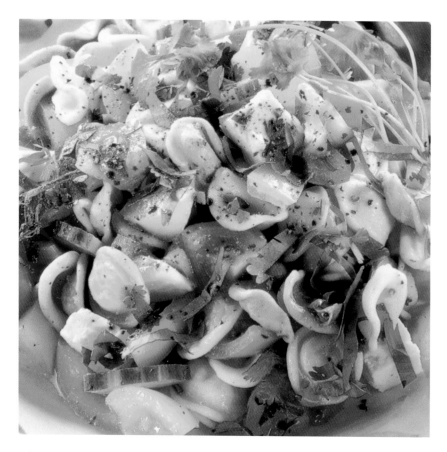

550 g fresh orecchiette (ears)

dash of olive oil

450 g red and yellow tomatoes, chopped

15 cm piece of cucumber chopped

175 g feta cheese, chopped

5 tbsp chopped fresh coriander

2 tbsp chopped fresh basil

FOR THE DRESSING

1 tbsp white wine vinegar

4 tbsp olive oil

2 garlic cloves, crushed

freshly ground black pepper

1 Bring a large saucepan of water to the boil and add the orecchiette with a dash of olive oil. Cook for about 5 minutes, stirring occasionally, until tender.

2 Drain and rinse under cold running water. Drain again and set aside.

3 Place the orecchiette in a large mixing bowl and add the remaining salad ingredients. Mix to combine.

4 To make the dressing, place all the ingredients in a screw-top jar and shake well. Pour the dressing over the salad and toss to coat.

5 Serve garnished with cherry tomatoes and coriander sprigs.

NUTRITIONAL VALUES

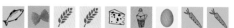

TRICOLOUR TOFU SALAD

SERVES **4**

Tofu replaces mozzarella in this popular Italian salad. Use the fullest-flavoured tomatoes that are in season – cherry, plum, vine or beef would be suitable.

100 ml extra virgin olive oil

2 tbsp balsamic vinegar

1 garlic clove, peeled and crushed

1 small shallot, peeled and very finely chopped

freshly ground black pepper

250 g firm tofu, sliced

2 red peppers

350 g tomatoes

1 ripe avocado

basil leaves, to garnish

warm focaccia bread to serve

1 Place the olive oil, vinegar, garlic, shallot and seasoning in a screw-top jar and shake until thouroughly mixed. Arrange the tofu slices in a shallow dish and pour over the dressing. Cover and chill for 2 hours.

2 Grill the peppers until the skins are scorched all over. Place in a bowl, cover and leave until cool enough to handle, then strip away the skins, deseed and cut into wedges.

3 Slice, halve or quarter the tomatoes according to size. Halve the avocado, remove the stone, peel and slice.

4 Arrange the tofu, tomatoes, peppers and avocado slices on a large serving dish. Spoon the dressing remaining in the dish over the mixture and sprinkle with the basil leaves. Serve at once with warm focaccia bread.

NUTRITIONAL VALUES

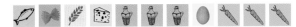

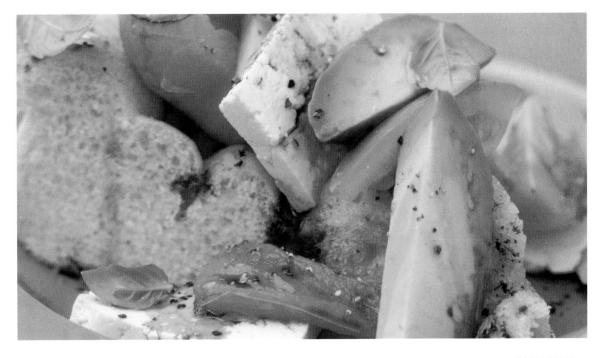

MICHAELMAS SALAD

SERVES **4**

This salad is very good with smoked salmon and with any herring dishes. It is also delicious on its own, accompanied with soda bread for a light lunch.

675 g freshly boiled beetroot

bunch of spring onions

bunch of french dill, chopped

2 tbsp chopped parsley

2 hard-boiled eggs, chopped

2 boiled potatoes, diced

olive oil

crushed garlic

lemon juice

1 Put the first six ingredients in a glass bowl. Dress with a vinaigrette made with the olive oil, garlic and lemon juice. As a general rule combine in the following proportions – $^1/_3$ lemon juice to $^2/_3$ olive oil – and add garlic to taste.

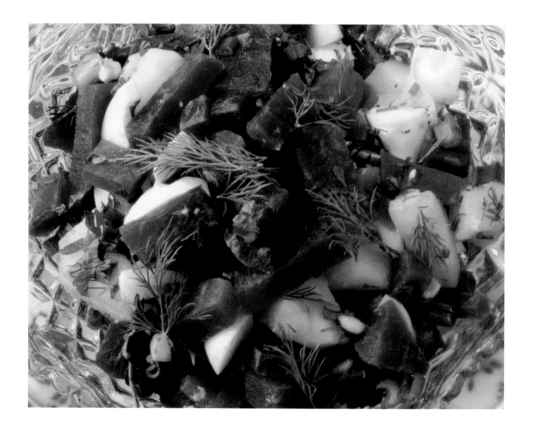

NUTRITIONAL VALUES

VEGETABLE GRATIN

SERVES **4**

A light and colourful vegetable dish that can be used as a snack, starter or even an accompaniment with a meal.

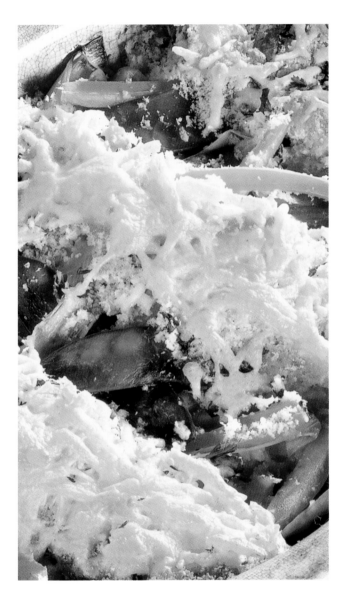

2 leeks, cut into strips lengthways

2 carrots, cut into sticks

75 g snow peas

150 g baby corn, halved

2 garlic cloves, minced

1 tbsp clear honey

1/2 tsp ground ginger

1/4 tsp freshly grated nutmeg

167 ml apple juice

167 ml vegetable broth

60 g fresh white bread crumbs

2 tbsp chopped fresh coriander

30 g shredded low-fat cheese

NUTRITIONAL VALUES

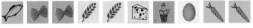

1 Place the vegetables in a large pan of boiling water and cook for 10 minutes.

2 Drain well and place in a shallow ovenproof dish. Mix together the garlic, honey, ginger, nutmeg, apple juice and broth, and pour over the vegetables.

3 Mix together the bread crumbs and coriander. Sprinkle over the vegetables to cover. Top with the cheese.

4 Bake in the oven at 200°C/gas mark 6 for 45 minutes or until golden brown. Serve immediately.

TOMATO SPAGHETTI WITH MUSHROOMS

SERVES **4 – 6**

For this dish you need to include at least one kind of dried mushroom as this will give the depth of flavour that is so typical of Italian mushroom-based dishes. Dried porcini keep well, and are an ingredient that no well-stocked kitchen should be without.

FOR THE DRESSING

15 g dried porcini mushrooms

3 tbsp olive oil

1 red onion, peeled and cut into
  wedges

3–6 smoked or regular garlic cloves,
  thinly sliced

125 g mushrooms, such as oyster or
  chanterelle, wiped and sliced

125 g button mushrooms, wiped and
  sliced

6 tbsp red wine

2 tbsp extra virgin olive oil

salt substitute (see page 15) and freshly
  ground black pepper

2 tbsp chopped fresh sage

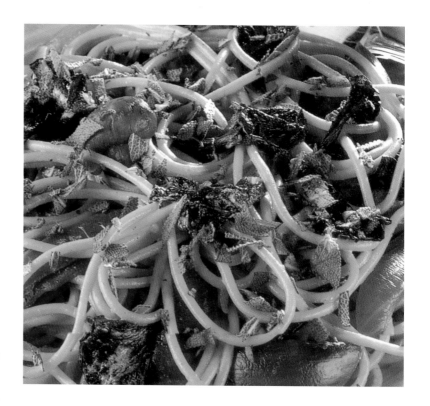

NUTRITIONAL VALUES

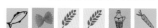

TO SERVE

450 g fresh tomato spaghetti

chopped fresh sage

1 Soak the porcini in warm water for about 20 minutes. Drain, reserving the soaking liquid, and chop the porcini.

2 Heat the oil in the pan and sauté the onion and garlic for 3 minutes. Add the chopped porcini, oyster or chanterelle and button mushrooms. Sauté for a further 5 minutes, stirring frequently.

3 Strain the porcini soaking liquid into the pan and add the red wine. Bring to the boil, then simmer for 5 minutes or until the mushrooms are just cooked and the liquid has been reduced by about a half. Stir in the extra virgin oil, season to taste, and add the sage. Cover with the lid, remove from the heat, and reserve.

4 Meanwhile, cook the tomato spaghetti in plenty of boiling water for 3 to 4 minutes or until firm to the bite. Drain and return to the pan. Add the mushrooms and sauce, and toss the ingredients lightly. Serve, garnished with the chopped fresh sage.

BEAN AND VEGETABLE PASTIES

SERVES **4**

Pasties are the traditional food of the mining community of Cornwall, southwest England. Originally made with shin of beef and root vegetables, the pasties had the miners' initials in pastry on them – not for garnish, but to show ownership. These bean and vegetable pasties make a good vegetarian alternative to the traditional meat pies of Cornwall.

50 g mung beans, soaked overnight

PASTRY

50 g olive oil

175 g fine wholewheat flour

pinch of salt substitute (see page 15)

1 onion finely chopped

100 g finely diced mixed root vegetables

50 g finely diced cheddar cheese

salt substitute (see page 15) and freshly ground
   black pepper

1 tbsp freshly chopped mixed herbs (optional)

1 Drain the beans and rinse them thoroughly under cold running water. Bring to the boil in a pan of fresh water, then simmer for 30 minutes, until tender. Drain and set aside until needed.

2 Preheat an oven to 200°C/gas mark 6. Prepare the pastry by blending the olive oil into the flour and salt substitute (see page 15). Add sufficient warm water to give a firm but workable dough, then knead lightly on a floured surface. Divide the dough into 4 and roll out into 6-inch diameter circles.

3 Mix the mung beans with all the remaining ingredients and divide the mixture between the pastry circles. Damp the edges with water, then draw the pastry together over the filling, pinching the edges together to seal them.

4 Place the pasties on a lightly oiled baking sheet. Cook in the preheated oven for 30–40 minutes, until the pastry is crisp. Serve hot or cold.

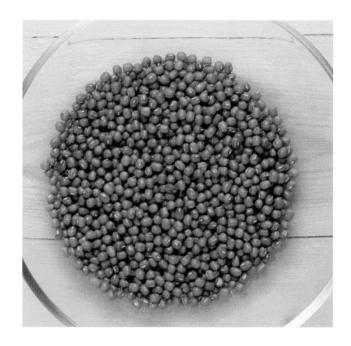

NUTRITIONAL VALUES

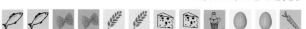

WILD RICE CASSEROLE

Wild rice is still something of a luxury for many of us, being very expensive to harvest in the traditional way – from swamp boats. It is not really a rice – more a grass seed – but that does not sound gastronomically correct! A cultivated wild rice is now available, more reasonably priced.

3 tbsp olive oil

1 onion, finely chopped

1 red pepper, chopped

150 g chopped mushrooms

100 g pecan nuts, roughly chopped

150 g wild rice

700 ml well-flavoured chicken or vegetable
   stock

4–5 tbsp freshly chopped parsley

freshly ground black pepper

freshly chopped parsley to garnish

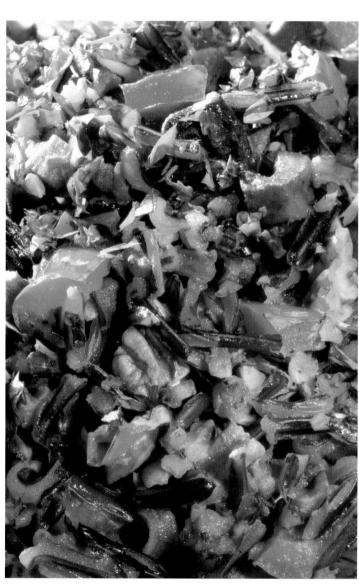

1 Preheat the oven to 160°C/gas mark 3. Heat the oil in a large flameproof casserole, then add the onion and pepper and cook slowly for about 5 minutes.

2 Stir in the mushrooms and pecans and continue cooking until the juices run from the mushrooms, then add the wild rice. Stir well, then pour in the stock.

3 Bring the casserole to the boil then add the parsley. Cover and bake in the preheated oven for 1¹/₄–1¹/₂ hours, until the rice has absorbed practically all the stock. Season to taste, then serve with a green salad.

NUTRITIONAL VALUES

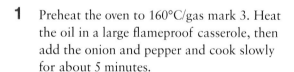

EASTERN PASTA SALAD

SERVES **4 – 6**

A traditional combination of mint and lemon makes this dish a salad for summer. Choose your favourite pasta shapes for this recipe and serve with warm pita bread to mop up the delicious dressing.

350 g dried pasta

dash of olive oil

400 g can chick peas, drained

4 tbsp chopped fresh mint

finely grated zest of 1 lemon

FOR THE DRESSING

3 garlic cloves, crushed

6 tbsp extra virgin olive oil

3 tbsp white wine vinegar

freshly squeezed juice of 1 lemon

freshly ground black pepper

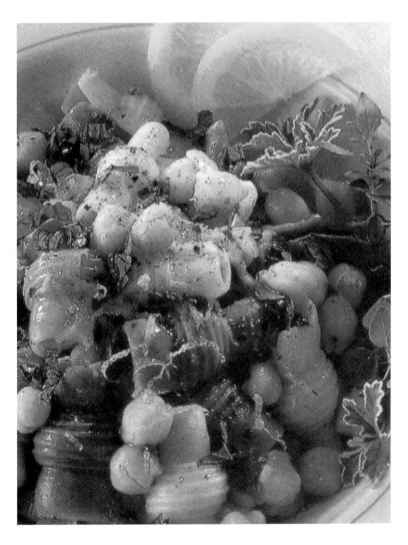

1 Bring a large saucepan of water to the boil and add the pasta with a dash of olive oil. Cook for about 10 minutes, stirring occasionally, until tender.

2 Drain and rinse under cold running water. Drain again and place in a large mixing bowl.

3 Add the chickpeas, mint and lemon zest to the pasta. Place all the dressing ingredients in a screw-top jar and shake well to mix.

4 Pour the dressing over the chickpea mixture and mix well to combine. Cover and chill for at least 30 minutes. Toss before serving.

NUTRITIONAL VALUES

SMOKED TROUT AND RASPBERRY SALAD WITH LINGONBERRY DRESSING

SERVES **4**

A very light, fruity and refreshing way to eat trout, making this an ideal dish for the summer.

250 ml low-fat crème fraîche

4 tbsp lingonberry preserve

juice of 1 lemon

pepper

2 bunches of rocket, washed thoroughly in cold water, and torn into bite-sized pieces

1 red onion, thinly sliced

1 whole smoked trout, about 350 g, picked off the bone and broken into bite-sized pieces

8 plum tomatoes, cut into quarters

125 g fresh raspberries

1 In a small bowl, combine low-fat crème fraîche, preserve, lemon juice and pepper.

2 In a medium bowl, toss rocket with red onion. Spread out on 4 plates. Arrange trout pieces, tomato pieces and raspberries on top. Add dressing.

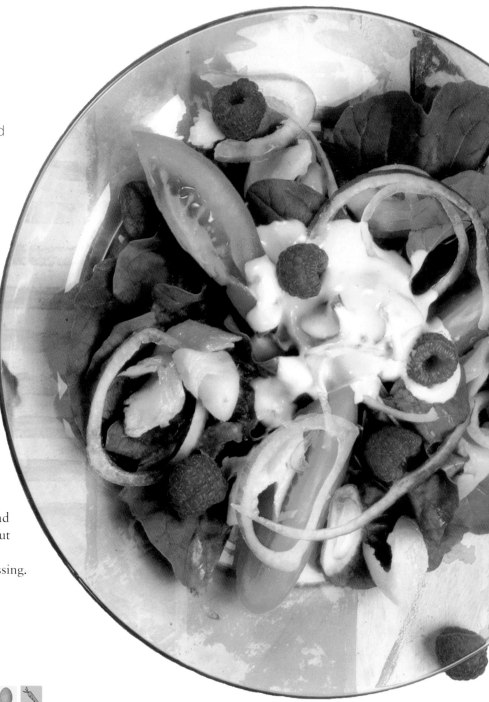

NUTRITIONAL VALUES

     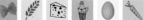

SQUASH AND COURGETTE TROUT

SERVES **4**

Trout are such versatile fish and yet they are so often just served with almonds and slightly burnt butter. A mixture of squash and courgette complements the oily fish, and a fruity orange sauce finishes the dish well.

4 tbsp olive oil

1 courgette, diced fine

225 g diced, cooked squash, such as crown
   prince

4 rainbow or brown trout, about 250–275 g each

grated rind and juice of 2 oranges

3 kaffir lime leaves, finely sliced

1–2 tbsp plain yoghurt

ground black pepper

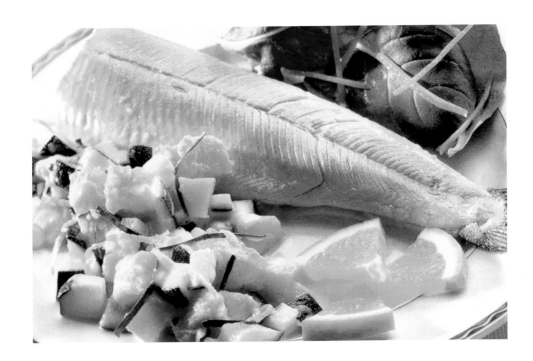

1 Heat the oil in a large frying pan, then add the diced courgette and squash. Cook for 3–4 minutes, until lightly browned, then scoop the vegetables out of the pan into an ovenproof dish, and keep warm.

2 Add a little extra oil to the pan, then add the trout and fry gently for 5–6 minutes on each side. You might have to cook just two at a time. Transfer them to a plate and keep warm in a very low oven while finishing the sauce.

3 Return the courgette and squash to the pan with the orange juice and sliced lime leaves. Cook for 1–2 minutes, then add the yoghurt.

4 Cook gently until the yoghurt has heated through, add the orange rind, and season. Serve the sauce spooned over the fish, with crusty granary rolls.

NUTRITIONAL VALUES

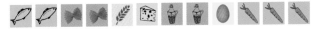

TUNA AND POTATO SALAD

SERVES **3 – 4**

In the Algarve and Madeira fresh tuna is prized and popular, but elsewhere (and even in those places) canned tuna is used for salads and appetizers such as this well-flavoured salad from Sesimbra, a quaint fishing village south of Lisbon.

NUTRITIONAL VALUES

350 g waxy potatoes

salt substitute (see page 15) and freshly ground
  pepper

3 tbsp olive oil

1 1/2 tbsp white wine vinegar

1/2 small onion, finely chopped

125 g canned tuna, flaked

1 hard-boiled egg white, sliced

1 small tomato, deseeded and
  chopped

1 1/2 tbsp chopped parsley

TO GARNISH

sliced tomato

sliced egg

parsley sprigs

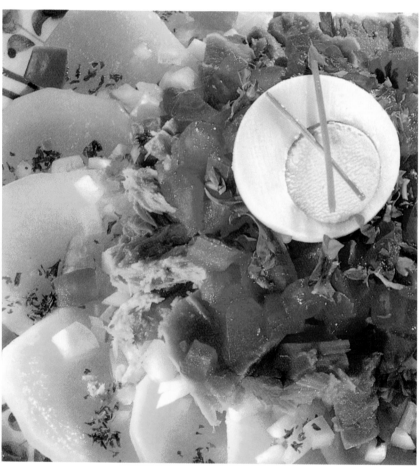

1 Cook the potatoes in boiling water for 10 minutes. Remove from the heat and leave to cool until tender, about 15 minutes. Drain, peel and slice thinly.

2 Whisk together the oil, vinegar and seasoning. Brush a little of this dressing over the bottom of a serving dish. Lay half the potato slices in the dish. Cover with half the onion, tuna, egg, tomato and parsley. Pour over the remaining dressing. Repeat with the remaining ingredients.

3 Cover and leave for at least 1 hour. Serve garnished with tomato, egg and parsley.

MINTY CRAB, PEAR AND PASTA SALAD

SERVES **4**

The dressing used in this recipe was found in an old recipe book. It has been updated using a flavoured vinegar and oil, and once you have tasted this it will quickly become a firm favourite.

FOR THE SALAD

225 g cooked fresh pasta, such as tri-coloured
   spaghetti

200 g white crab meat, flaked

2 oranges, peeled and cut into sections

2 pink grapefruit, peeled and cut into sections

2 tbsp chopped fresh mint

65 g pecan halves

FOR THE DRESSING

2 ripe pears

100 ml walnut oil

4 tbsp extra virgin olive oil

1 tbsp orange or raspberry vinegar

ground black pepper

1 Place the cooked pasta in a bowl and add the flaked crab meat, orange and grapefruit sections, chopped mint and pecan halves. Toss lightly and spoon into a serving bowl.

2 For the dressing, peel and core the pears, then place in a food processor. Gradually blend the pears with the walnut oil and then the olive oil. Add the vinegar with seasoning and blend for 30 seconds or until smooth. Pour over the salad, toss lightly and serve.

NUTRITIONAL VALUES

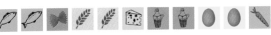

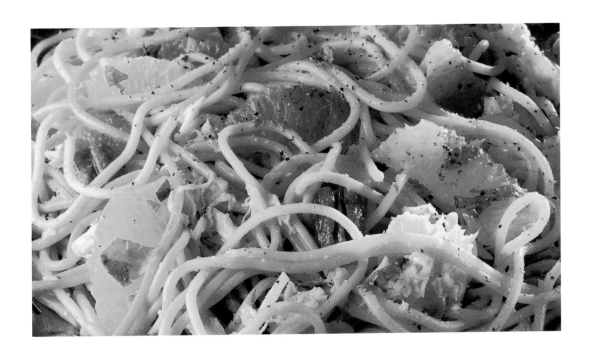

CRAB BALLS WITH SWEET LIME SAUCE

SERVES **4**

This recipe is quick and convenient, using canned white crab meat although if you can get fresh white crab meat, use that. The lime sauce is only very slightly sweet, so prepare to have your taste buds roused!

225 g can white crab meat, drained and
squeezed dry

75 g fresh wholewheat breadcrumbs

4 spring onions, trimmed and very finely chopped

freshly ground black pepper

freshly grated nutmeg

1 large egg, beaten

75 ml olive oil for frying

SAUCE

grated rind and juice of 2 limes

1 tbsp demerara sugar

1 red chilli, seeded and very finely chopped

NUTRITIONAL VALUES

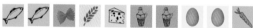

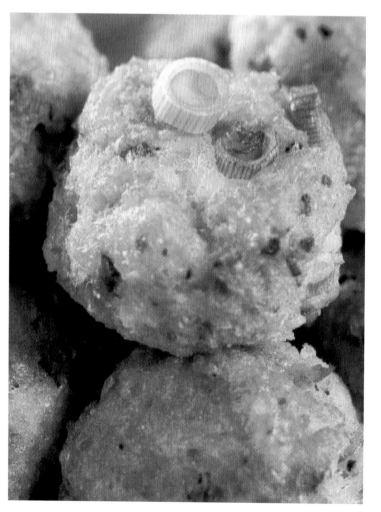

1   Mix all the ingredients for the sauce together and set aside until needed.

2   Mix the crab meat with the breadcrumbs and spring onions then season with pepper and nutmeg. Add the egg and blend the mixture together. Shape into 20 walnut-sized pieces – you may have to flour your hands to do this.

3   Heat the oil in a frying pan and add the crab balls. Fry them for about 4–5 minutes until evenly browned all over, turning occasionally. Drain on paper towels, then serve immediately with the lime sauce for dipping.

MEDITERRANEAN CHICKEN SALAD

SERVES **6**

Fresh herbs make all the difference in this summer salad. For a change, substitute flaked tuna fish for the ham and fresh tarragon for the basil.

175 g cooked chicken

100–125 g cooked ham

175 g French beans or green (string or snap) beans, lightly cooked

175 g new potatoes, cooked

4 plum or cherry tomatoes (yellow or red variety)

$1/2$ cucumber, peeled

12 black olives

1 tbsp each freshly chopped basil, parsley, and chives

4 tbsp olive oil

1 tbsp white wine vinegar

1 tbsp lemon juice

pinch dry mustard powder

pinch cayenne

freshly ground black pepper

GARNISH

6 anchovies

fresh herb sprigs

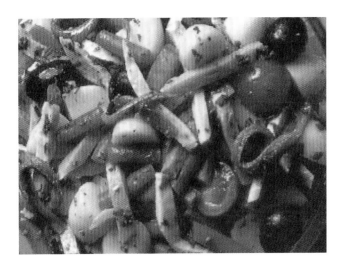

1   Cut the chicken and ham into neat strips. Cut the beans into 2.5 cm lengths and the potatoes into small chunks. Place in a large bowl.

2   Halve or slice the tomatoes, depending on size. Cut the cucumber in half lengthways, scoop out and discard the seeds, then cut the flesh into matchsticks. Add to the bowl.

3   Fold these ingredients together carefully, together with the freshly chopped herbs and olives.

4   In a screw-top jar, shake together the olive oil, wine vinegar, lemon juice, mustard powder, cayenne and seasonings until well blended. Pour over the chicken salad.

5   Spoon the salad into a glass serving dish. Garnish the top with fresh anchovies and sprigs of herbs. Chill for at least 1 hour before serving to allow the flavours to develop.

NUTRITIONAL VALUES

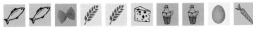

STUFFED GREEN PEPPERS WITH CHILLI MINCE

SERVES **6**

A spicy starter or light meal to warm the tastebuds, with a crispy cheesy topping.

1 onion, finely chopped

60 ml olive oil

3 large or 6 small green peppers

500 g minced (ground) beef or pork

2 tsp garlic, crushed

6 red chillies, finely chopped

1/2 tsp oregano

1 bay leaf

500 ml water

pepper

2 tsp tomato purée

1 tsp basil, chopped

2 beef (large) tomatoes, peeled and chopped

225 g can kidney beans

100 g grated manchego cheese

1 To prepare the filling gently cook the onion in the oil. Add the meat, garlic, chillies, oregano, bay leaf, water, pepper, tomato purée and basil, and cook, stirring, until it reaches the boil.

2 Lower heat and simmer for 45 minutes, stirring occasionally. Add the beans and tomato, season to taste and bring to the boil. Remove from heat.

3 To prepare the peppers, remove the stalks. Plunge into boiling water and simmer for 5 minutes. Immediately cool in cold water and drain.

4 If peppers are large, cut in half lengthways, and remove seeds. Fill with the meat mixture. Sprinkle with cheese and bake at 200°C/gas mark 6, until the cheese melts.

5 If the peppers are small, cut off the tops and keep them aside. Carefully remove the seeds and core. Trim base so that the pepper will sit squarely, without making a hole in it. Fill with the meat mixture and sprinkle with cheese. Place on a baking tray with the top next to it to heat up. When cheese is melted, replace top and serve.

NUTRITIONAL VALUES

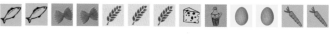

STARTERS

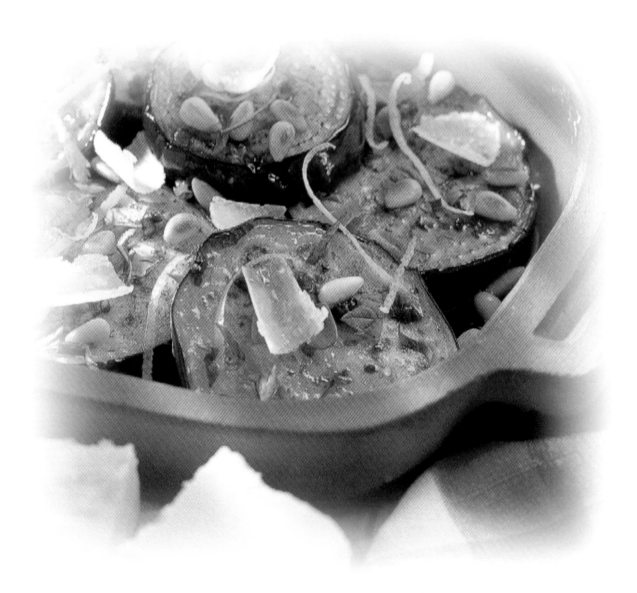

PIQUANT TOMATO SORBET

SERVES **4 – 6**

A lovely cool starter or can be eaten just as a savoury snack, especially suitable for a hot summer's day.

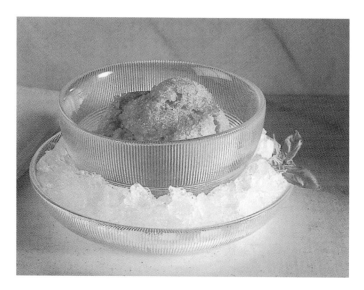

500 g ripe tomatoes, skinned and chopped

1 onion, chopped

2 garlic cloves, crushed

225 g can tomatoes

1 tbsp fresh basil, chopped

1 tbsp Worcestershire sauce

4–5 drops Tabasco

2 tbsp tomato purée

pepper

2 tbsp lemon juice

1 tsp powdered gelatine

1 egg white

TO GARNISH

basil leaves

NUTRITIONAL VALUES

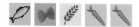

1 Peel the tomatoes by pricking and placing them in a bowl with 700 ml boiling water. Microwave on high for 30 seconds. Drain and plunge in cold water. Peel the skins off using a knife.

2 Place the tomatoes, onion and garlic in a casserole dish, cover and microwave on high for 6 minutes. Add the canned tomatoes and basil, re-cover and microwave on high for 5 minutes.

3 Add the Worcestershire sauce, Tabasco, tomato purée and seasoning and stir well.

4 Place the lemon juice in a small bowl and sprinkle the gelatine over. Leave for 5 minutes then microwave on high for 20–30 seconds to dissolve.

5 Sieve the tomato mix into a bowl and stir in the gelatine. Place in a shallow freezer proof container and freeze until slushy.

6 Whisk the egg white until stiff, then whisk the tomato mix and fold in the egg white. If wished place the dishes on a bed of crushed ice to serve.

SMOKED HADDOCK
AND BROAD BEAN CHOWDER

SERVES **4**

This soup is definitely better if you remove the broad beans from their tough outer skins. It may be a little time-consuming but it is well worth the effort.

2 tbsp olive oil

1 medium onion, peeled and chopped

350 g new potatoes, scrubbed and diced

1 tbsp flour

450 ml vegetable stock

300 g smoked haddock fillet, skinned and diced

150 ml semi-skimmed milk

freshly ground black pepper

75 g sweetcorn kernels, thawed if frozen

100 g broad beans, removed from skins, thawed if
    frozen

1 tbsp freshly chopped parsley

2–3 tbsp low-fat sour cream

crusty bread to serve

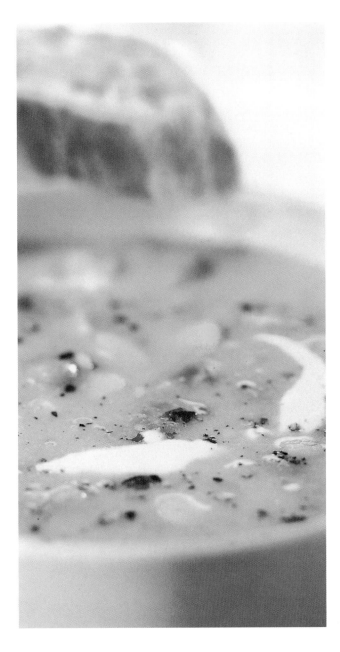

1   Preheat the cooker on high. Pour oil in a pan; then sauté the onion and potatoes for 3 minutes, stirring frequently. Sprinkle in the flour and cook for 2 minutes; then take the pan off the heat. Gradually stir in the stock and bring to the boil. Add the diced, smoked haddock with the milk and a little freshly ground black pepper.

2   Spoon or pour into the cooking pot, cover and reduce the temperature to low. Cook for 4 hours. Mix the corn and broad beans together then add to the cooking pot and continue to cook for an additional 1–2 hours.

3   Stir in the chopped parsley, adjust the seasoning and serve with spoonfuls of low-fat sour cream and chunks of crusty bread.

NUTRITIONAL VALUES

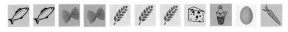

COURGETTE AND MINT SOUP

SERVES **4**

This delicate soup has a silky texture and a hint of mint.

900 ml vegetable stock

1 onion, chopped

1 garlic clove, minced

3 courgettes, shredded

1 large potato, scrubbed and chopped

1 tbsp chopped fresh mint

freshly ground black pepper

150 ml low-fat plain yoghurt

TO GARNISH

mint sprigs and courgette strips

1 Put half of the vegetable stock in a large pan, add the onion and garlic, and cook for 5 minutes over a gentle heat until the onion softens.

2 Add the shredded courgettes, potato and remaining stock. Stir in the mint and cook over a gentle heat for 20 minutes or until the potato is cooked.

3 Transfer the soup to a food processor and blend for 10 seconds, until almost smooth. Turn the soup into a bowl, season and stir in the yoghurt. Cover and chill for 2 hours.

4 Spoon the soup into individual serving bowls or a soup tureen, garnish and serve.

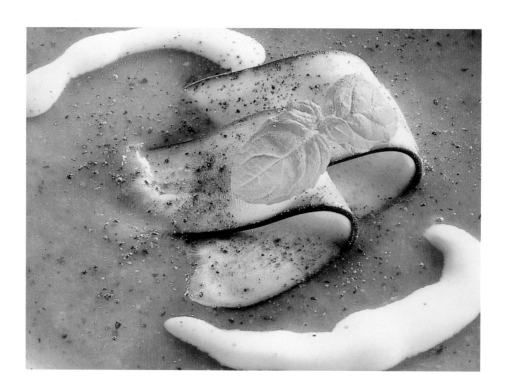

NUTRITIONAL VALUES

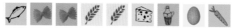

CLASSIC GREEK VEGETABLE SOUP

SERVES 6–8

Serve this classic Greek soup with freshly baked olive bread (eliopitta) for a truly authentic flavour of Greece.

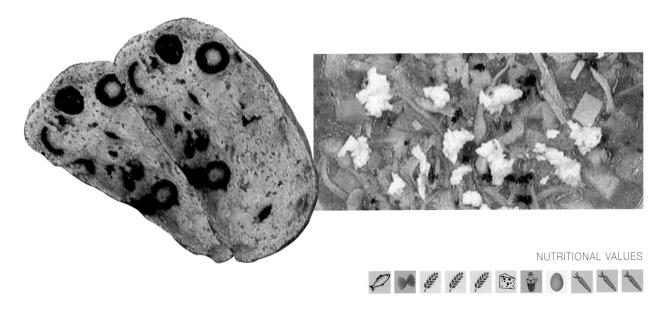

NUTRITIONAL VALUES

125 ml olive oil

2 garlic cloves, crushed

2 onions, finely chopped

375 g finely shredded cabbage

3 carrots, chopped

3 celery sticks, chopped

2 large potatoes, peeled and diced

1.5 litre vegetable stock or water

4 tomatoes, peeled, deseeded, and chopped

freshly ground black pepper, to taste

4 tbsp chopped fresh parsley

50 g feta or kefalotyri cheese, grated

1 Heat the olive oil in a large saucepan and add the garlic and onion. Cook for 5 minutes, until the onion is softened but not coloured. Add the cabbage and continue to cook for another 3–4 minutes.

2 Add the carrots and celery to the saucepan, stir and cook for a further 5 minutes. Add the potatoes, stir and cook gently for another 5 minutes, until the vegetables are softened.

3 Pour in the vegetable stock or water and stir well. Increase the heat to bring the soup to a boil. Cover and simmer for 12–15 minutes. Add the tomato and season to taste with freshly ground black pepper. Re-cover and gently simmer the soup for about 1 hour. Stir in the parsley just before the end of the cooking time. Serve sprinkled with grated cheese.

PASTA BEAN SOUP

SERVES **4 – 6**

A nutritious meal in itself – low-fat and full of protein. Serve with warm, crusty garlic bread.

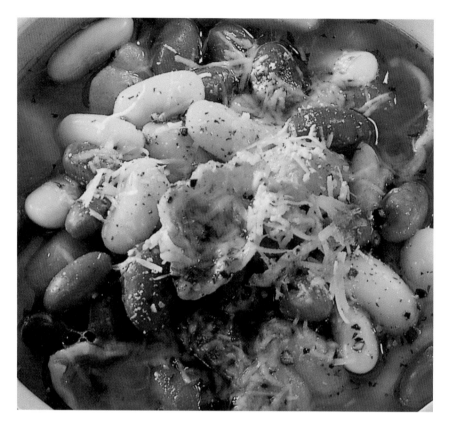

2 tbsp olive oil

3 garlic cloves, minced

4 tbsp chopped fresh parsley

150 g dried wholewheat gnocchi
  piccoli (shells)

1.75 litre vegetable stock

3 tbsp vegetable or tomato purée

400 g can mixed beans, such as
  borlotti, kidney, cannellini, etc,
  drained

freshly ground black pepper

TO SERVE

freshly grated Parmesan cheese

1 Heat the olive oil in a large pan and sauté the garlic with the chopped parsley for about 2 minutes. Add the gnocchi piccoli and cook for 1 to 2 minutes, stirring constantly.

2 Pour in the vegetable stock and add the vegetable or tomato purée. Bring to the boil, reduce the heat, then simmer for about 10 minutes, stirring occasionally, until the pasta is tender.

3 Add the beans and season with freshly ground black pepper. Continue to cook for a further 5 minutes, then serve with a little freshly grated Parmesan cheese.

NUTRITIONAL VALUES

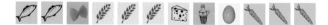

SORREL SOUP

SERVES **4**

This is a traditional soup from Ireland, which is still very popular today. It is high in fibre and antioxidants, but is also high in flavour. It is an ideal dish to serve on a cold winter's day.

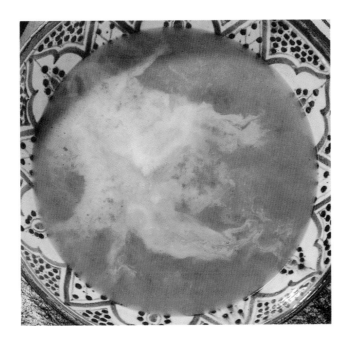

NUTRITIONAL VALUES

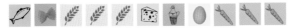

4 tbsp olive oil

1 large Spanish onion

4 garlic cloves

450 g sorrel

2.25 litre chicken stock

2 tbsp medium oatmeal

freshly ground black pepper

150 ml low-fat crème fraîche

1 Heat the oil in a pan. Chop the onion and garlic and soften them in the oil. Wash and tear the sorrel, then add to the onions, oil and garlic. Add the stock and bring to the boil.

2 Scatter the oatmeal and stir until cooked. Season the soup to taste and simmer for about 1 hour.

3 Serve in warm bowls with a dollop of crème fraîche.

LENTIL AND SQUASH BROTH

SERVES **6**

This broth is ideal to serve when the weather is beginning to turn cold or a bowl of comfort food is required. Ideal for cooking in a slow cooker.

2 tbsp olive oil

1 small butternut or harlequin squash, about 450 g, peeled, deseeded and chopped

3 celery stalks, trimmed and chopped

1 tsp dried, crushed chillies

100 g red lentils

2 tbsp tomato purée

1.2 litre vegetable stock

freshly ground black pepper

TO GARNISH

fresh coriander sprigs

freshly grated hard cheese, such as Cheddar or Monterey Jack

1 Preheat the cooker on high. Heat the oil in a large pan and sauté the squash, chopped celery, onion and crushed chillies for 5 minutes. Add the lentils and cook, stirring, for 2 more minutes.

2 Blend the tomato purée with a little of the stock, add to the pan, stir, then pour in the remaining stock. Bring to the boil, add a little seasoning, then pour or spoon into the cooking pot.

3 Reduce the temperature to low, cover and cook for 6–8 hours. When ready to serve, blend the soup until smooth and add seasoning. Reheat if necessary and serve, sprinkling with a little cheese and garnishing with fresh coriander sprigs.

NUTRITIONAL VALUES

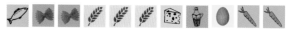

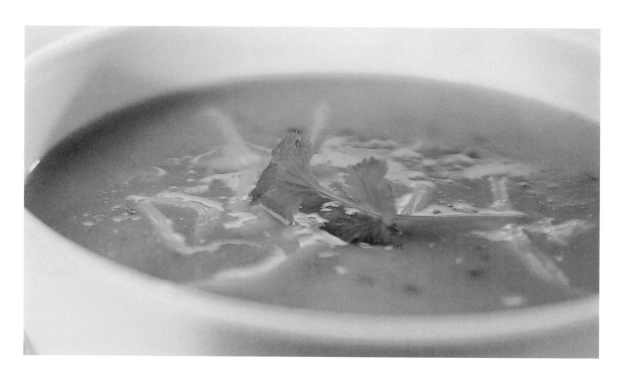

FISH SOUP

SERVES **4**

This fish soup is very good served with croutons, and may be made with any firm white fish. For another variation, add a pinch of curry powder instead of the paprika at the end.

450–675 g mixed vegetables, finely chopped
    (carrots, shallots, onions, fennel, leeks, celery,
    tomatoes, potatoes)

4 tbsp olive oil

1.2 litre fish stock

bay leaf and fresh herbs

2 garlic cloves

675–900 g firm white fish

1 glass dry white wine

2 tbsp chopped parsley

150 ml crème fraîche

pepper and paprika

NUTRITIONAL VALUES

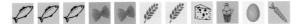

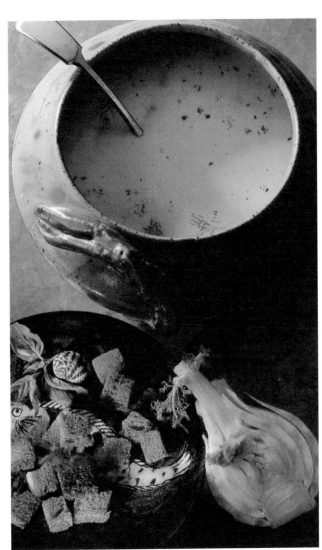

1 Toss the vegetables in 2 tablespoons of the oil. Add the stock, herbs, and garlic, and simmer until the vegetables are cooked.

2 Cut the fish into chunks and poach gently in the wine. Remove the fish from the liquid, whisk in the remaining oil and add to the stock and vegetables. Sprinkle in the chopped parsley, flake the fish and add to the soup.

3 Just before serving, add the crème fraîche and heat to just below boiling point. Do not boil. Season, and add a pinch of paprika in the bowls.

CORN CHOWDER

SERVES **4**

A classic chowder never loses its appeal. Prepare in advance and freeze in convenient portion sizes for ease.

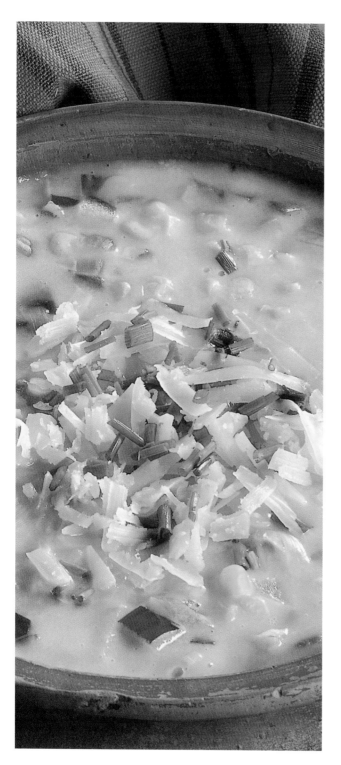

275 g drained, canned corn kernels

600 g vegetable broth

1 red onion, diced

1 green pepper, seeded and diced

600 ml skimmed milk

2 tbsp cornflour

187 g low-fat Cheddar or Edam cheese, shredded

1 tbsp fresh snipped chives

ground black pepper

TO GARNISH

snipped chives

NUTRITIONAL VALUES

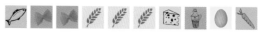

1   Place the corn, broth, onion and pepper in a pan. Blend 4 tablespoons of skimmed milk with the cornflour to form a paste.

2   Bring the pan contents to a boil, reduce the heat, and simmer for 20 minutes. Add the milk and cornflour paste and bring to the boil, stirring until thickened.

3   Stir in the cheese and chives and season. Heat until the cheese has melted, garnish, and serve.

VEGETABLE AND FRESH CORIANDER SOUP

SERVES **4 – 6**

A light, fresh-tasting soup that is ideal either as a starter or as a light lunch.

1 litre vegetable stock

100 g dried pasta (any shape)

dash of olive oil

2 carrots, thinly sliced

100 g frozen peas

6 tbsp chopped fresh coriander

freshly ground black pepper

TO SERVE

grated cheese, optional

NUTRITIONAL VALUES

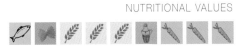

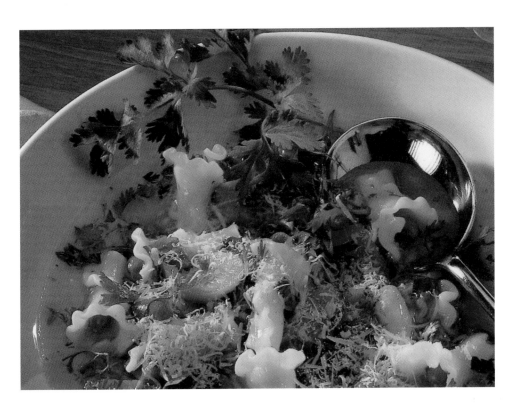

1 Bring the vegetable stock to the boil in a large saucepan and add the pasta with a dash of olive oil. Cook for about 5 minutes, stirring occasionally, then add the sliced carrots.

2 Cook for 5 minutes, then add the peas and coriander. Season with the freshly ground black pepper, and simmer gently for about 10 minutes, stirring occasionally, until the pasta and carrots are tender. Serve the soup with finely grated cheese, if wished.

BUTTERNUT AND ORANGE SOUP

SERVES **4 – 6**

This is a wonderful combination of flavours and will quickly establish itself as a family favourite. Do not boil the soup after adding the orange juice or the flavour will become slightly tainted.

NUTRITIONAL VALUES

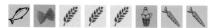

1 Cook the onion in the oil until softened but not browned, then add the prepared squash and cook slowly for 5 minutes, stirring occasionally. Stir in the grated orange rind then add the broth, bay leaves and seasonings. Bring the soup to the boil, then cover and simmer for 40 minutes, until the squash is tender and cooked through.

2 Allow the soup to cool slightly, remove the bay leaves, then purée in a blender or food processor until smooth. Rinse the pan and return the soup to it, adding the orange juice. Reheat the soup slowly – do not let it boil – then season to taste. Add the freshly chopped parsley just before serving.

1 onion, chopped

2 tbsp olive oil

1–2 butternut squashes, weighing about 900 g, peeled and diced

grated rind and juice of 2 oranges

1.5 litre well-flavoured vegetable stock

freshly ground black pepper

2 bay leaves

freshly grated nutmeg

TO GARNISH

2 tbsp freshly chopped parsley

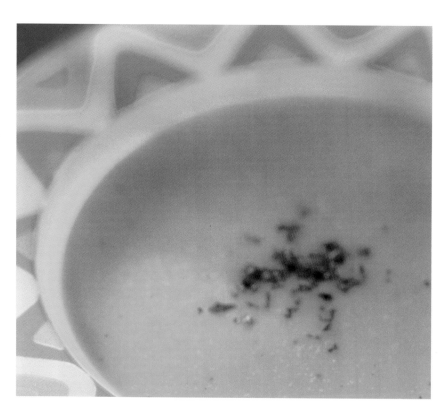

ROASTED TOMATO TARTLETS

SERVES **6**

This is a wonderful dish to make when home-grown tomatoes are plentiful and full of flavour. Add a few olives to the filling if you wish – they look attractive, but if the tomatoes are ripe and flavourful, they are not necessary.

3 onions, sliced finely

2 cloves garlic, halved

3 tbsp fruity olive oil

3–4 sprigs fresh thyme

2 bay leaves

4–5 large tomatoes, sliced

freshly ground black pepper

FOR THE DOUGH

250 g fine wholewheat flour

40 g sesame seeds

1/2 tsp salt substitute (see page 15)

1 large egg, beaten

75 ml olive oil

3–4 tbsp water

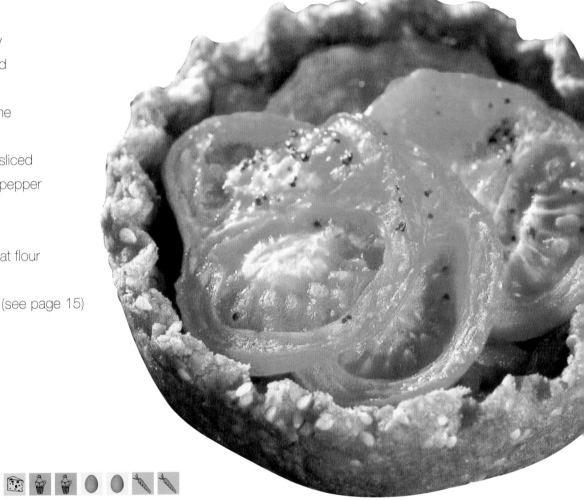

NUTRITIONAL VALUES

1 Mix together the flour, sesame seeds and salt substitute, then make a well in the centre. Add the egg and olive oil and mix to a soft dough, adding water as neessary. Divide the mixture into 6 and shape to line six 10 cm individual tart tins – this is more of a dough than a pastry and is easiest to mould into shape with your fingers. Chill the tart shells for at least 30 minutes while preparing the filling.

2 Cook the onions and garlic in the olive oil with the thyme and bay leaves for 30–40 minutes, until

well softened and reduced. Season to taste with salt and pepper, then remove the herbs.

3 Preheat the oven to 220°C/gas mark 7. Fill the tart shells with the onion mixture then top with the tomatoes, overlapping the slices and brushing them lightly with olive oil. Season well with the salt substitute and pepper, then bake in the preheated oven for 20–25 minutes, until the dough is crisp and the tomatoes are just starting to blacken. Serve hot or cold with a small, leafy salad.

BAKED STUFFED SWEET PEPPERS

SERVES **4**

When buying the sweet peppers, choose squat round ones that still stand upright. Choose green, red, yellow or orange peppers, or even a mixture.

4 even-sized sweet peppers

2 tbsp olive oil

1 small onion, finely chopped

125 g long grain rice

50 g button mushrooms, chopped

450 g chicken stock (broth)

4 tbsp tomato purée

2 tbsp fresh basil, chopped

freshly ground black pepper

4–6 chicken livers, chopped

2 tbsp pinenuts, toasted

2 tbsp finely grated Parmesan cheese

TO GARNISH

fresh basil leaves

NUTRITIONAL VALUES

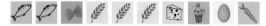

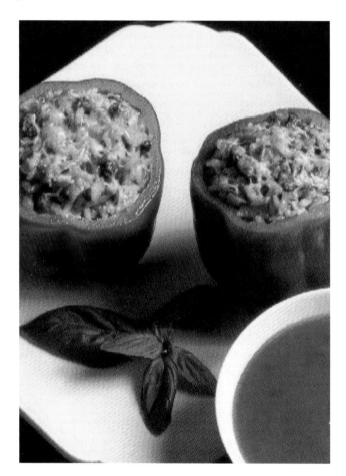

1 Cut the tops off the peppers and remove the cores and seeds. Put the peppers in a basin, cover with boiling water and allow to stand for 5 minutes. Drain thoroughly and set aside.

2 Heat half the oil in a large pan and sauté the onion until softened. Stir in the rice and mushrooms and cook for a further minute; add the stock (broth), bring to the boil and simmer, covered, for 15 minutes, until the rice is just tender and the stock absorbed.

3 Stir in the tomato purée and the freshly chopped basil. Season to taste.

4 Heat the remaining oil and sauté the chicken livers until lightly browned. Stir into the rice with the pinenuts.

5 Spoon the mixture into the peppers and sprinkle them with the cheese.

6 Arrange the peppers in an ovenproof dish. Pour a little water into the dish (just enough to cover its base) and cook for 35 minutes or until the peppers are tender. Serve hot, garnished with fresh basil leaves.

MANGETOUT SALAD

SERVES **4**

This brightly-coloured starter is a great beginning to any meal, and can be served as a light snack too. If you are unable to get hold of fresh mangetout, it is perfectly acceptable to use frozen.

100 g fresh shelled or frozen broad beans

2 tbsp lemon juice

175 g mangetout, trimmed

2 tbsp sesame seeds

3 tbsp olive oil

2 tsp soy sauce

freshly ground black pepper

6 baby tomatoes, quartered

1 small red pepper, deseeded and finely chopped

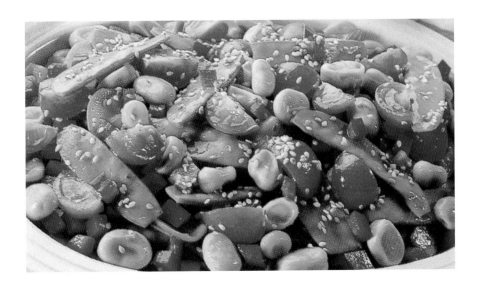

1 Place the broad beans in a casserole dish and add 1 tablespoon lemon juice and 4 tablespoons water. Cover and microwave on high for 5–7 minutes, or until tender. Stir after 3 minutes. Drain, refresh under cold running water and drain again.

2 Place the mangetout in a shallow dish with 3 tablespoons water. Cover and microwave on high for 2 minutes. Drain, refresh under cold running water and drain again.

3 Place the sesame seeds in a shallow heatproof dish and microwave on high for 6–8 minutes or until lightly browned. Stir 2–3 times. Leave to cool.

4 Place the olive oil in a small bowl and beat in the remaining lemon juice, soy sauce and seasoning.

5 Combine the beans, mangetout, tomatoes and pepper. Pour over the dressing and toss to coat.

6 Serve in 1 large or 4 small individual serving dishes, sprinkled with sesame seeds.

NUTRITIONAL VALUES

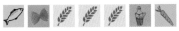

COUNTRY GRILLED AUBERGINE

SERVES **4**

An Italian-style salad of cooked aubergine slices marinated in oil and mint and finished with toasted pinenuts and parmesan.

1 large aubergine, thickly sliced

olive oil, for brushing

50 g pinenuts, toasted

2 tbsp chopped fresh parsley

grated zest of 1 lemon

shaved Parmesan cheese

MARINADE

125 g olive oil

1 garlic clove, crushed

12 large basil leaves, roughly torn

1 tbsp chopped fresh mint

freshly ground black pepper

1 tbsp balsamic vinegar

1 Preheat the grill or griddlepan until very hot, then add the aubergine slices. Brush generously with olive oil, then grill or griddle until browned on both sides.

2 Mix together the ingredients for the marinade in a shallow dish. Add the aubergine slices and turn them in the mixture. Leave for 1–2 hours, then stir in the pinenuts. Serve at room temperature, sprinkled with parsley, lemon zest and Parmesan, with fresh crusty bread.

NUTRITIONAL VALUES

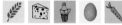

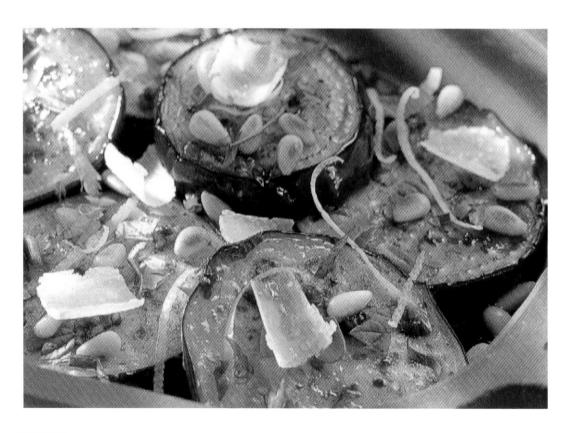

GRILLED VEGETABLES

SERVES **4**

These vegetables are great served on the side or as a meal in themselves with ciabatta or other breads to mop up the juices.

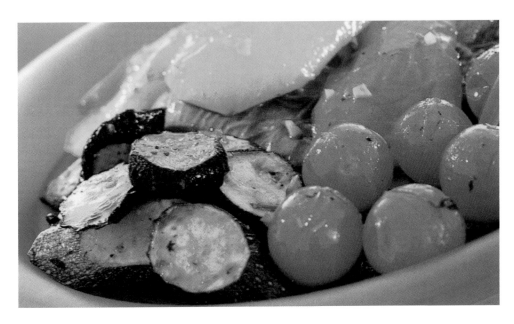

3 courgette, cut into 0.6 cm slices

1 red pepper, cut into wide wedges or halves

1 yellow and 1 green pepper, cut into quarters

3 tbsp extra virgin olive oil

5 garlic cloves, chopped

juice of ¹/₂ lemon or 1 tbsp balsamic vinegar or
white wine vinegar

14–20 cherry tomatoes

bamboo skewers, soaked in cold water for 30
minutes, or metal skewers

salt substitute (see page 15) and ground black
pepper

2–3 tbsp pesto or basil, finely chopped and puréed
with a little garlic and olive oil

1 Combine the courgette and peppers with the olive oil, garlic, and lemon or vinegar. Marinate for about 30 minutes if possible.

2 Meanwhile, thread the cherry tomatoes onto the skewers. Remove the courgette and peppers from the marinade, saving the marinade to dress the vegetables afterwards.

3 Grill the vegetables over a medium–high heat until lightly charred and brown in places and tender all the way through. Remove from the grill and return to the marinade. Let stand until the vegetables are cool enough to handle.

4 Meanwhile, grill the cherry tomatoes for about 5 minutes on each side or until slightly browned. Remove from the grill.

5 Dice the courgette and peppers, and slice the tomatoes. Season, combine the juices with the pesto or basil, pour over the vegetables and serve.

NUTRITIONAL VALUES

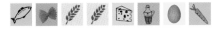

CREAMY GARLIC MUSHROOMS

SERVES **4**

Wonderful as a starter, but they also make perfect baked potato fillers!

2 tbsp olive oil

1 large garlic clove, crushed

2 spring onions, chopped

freshly ground black pepper

750 g button mushrooms

188 g low-fat cream cheese

TO GARNISH

a little parsley, chopped

NUTRITIONAL VALUES

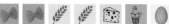

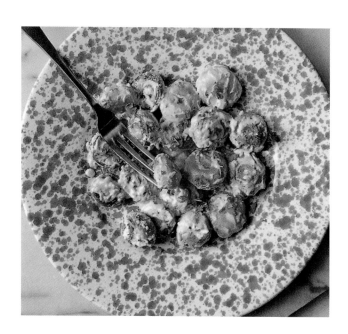

1 Heat the oil in a large frying pan. Add the garlic, onions and seasoning, and cook for 2 minutes. Then add all the mushrooms and toss them over high heat for a couple of minutes, until they are hot. Do not cook the mushrooms until their juices run as they will be too watery.

2 Make a clearing in the middle of the mushrooms, add the low-fat cream cheese and stir it in for a few seconds, until it begins to soften. Gradually mix all the mushrooms with the cheese until they are evenly coated.

3 Divide among individual plates or dishes and top with a little parsley, if liked. Serve at once with warmed wholewheat bread or toast.

4 Alternatively, transfer the mushrooms to a bowl, cool, then cover and chill them briefly before serving.

SOUSED HERRINGS WITH LOW-FAT SOUR CREAM

SERVES **4 – 6**

These can be eaten with or without the low-fat sour cream, and are also nice served with thick crusty wholemeal bread.

1 Preheat the oven to 170°C/gas mark 3. Wash the herring fillets and pat them dry with kitchen paper.

2 Place some of the thinly sliced onion, a bay leaf, and three whole peppercorns on each fish. Roll up the herrings with the tail-end away from you. Place in an ovenproof dish and cover with the vinegar and water mixture.

3 Place in a moderate oven until the herrings are cooked – about 20 minutes. Let the fish cool in the liquid for several hours or overnight.

4 Serve cold with a spoonful of the low-fat sours cream garnished with chopped dill.

6 fresh herring fillets

1 large Spanish onion, thinly sliced

6 bay leaves

18 whole black peppercorns

300 ml red wine vinegar mixed with water

300 ml low-fat sour cream

fresh dill, chopped

NUTRITIONAL VALUES

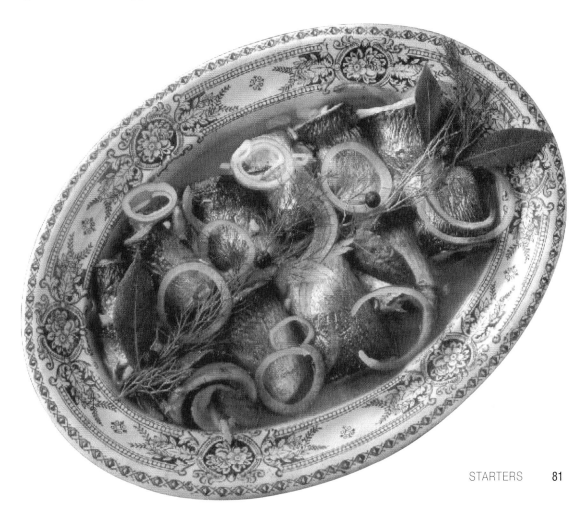

BLACKENED TUNA WITH STRAWBERRIES

SERVES **2**

An interesting combination of savoury and sweet, best served up on a bed of crispy green lettuce.

60 g unsalted butter

5–6 large strawberries, hulled and cut into thirds

$1/2$ tsp ground cumin

$1/2$ tsp ground cinnamon

$1/2$ tsp ground marjoram

$1/2$ tsp ground cayenne pepper

freshly ground black pepper

2 x 250 g tuna steaks

4 tbsp groundnut oil

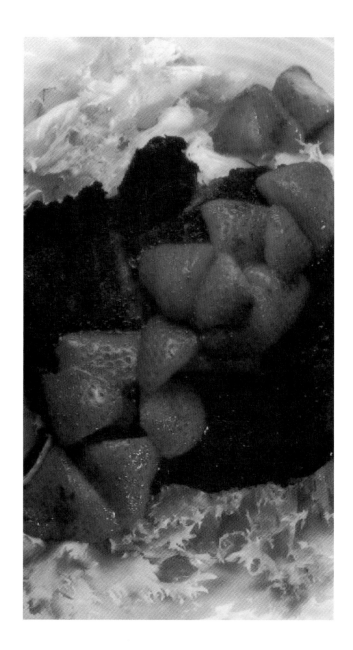

1 In a small frying pan over a low heat, melt the butter and add the strawberries. Sauté the strawberries for 3 minutes, until soft. Set aside.

2 Mix together the cumin, cinnamon, marjoram, cayenne pepper and pepper. Season generously with the mixture.

3 In a small cast-iron frying pan, heat the groundnut oil over high heat. Sear the fish until black, about 3–4 minutes. Turn over and blacken the other side, another 2–3 minutes. (This will produce a lot of smoke.)

4 Garnish the tuna with strawberries and serve.

NUTRITIONAL VALUES

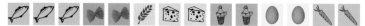

MAIN COURSES

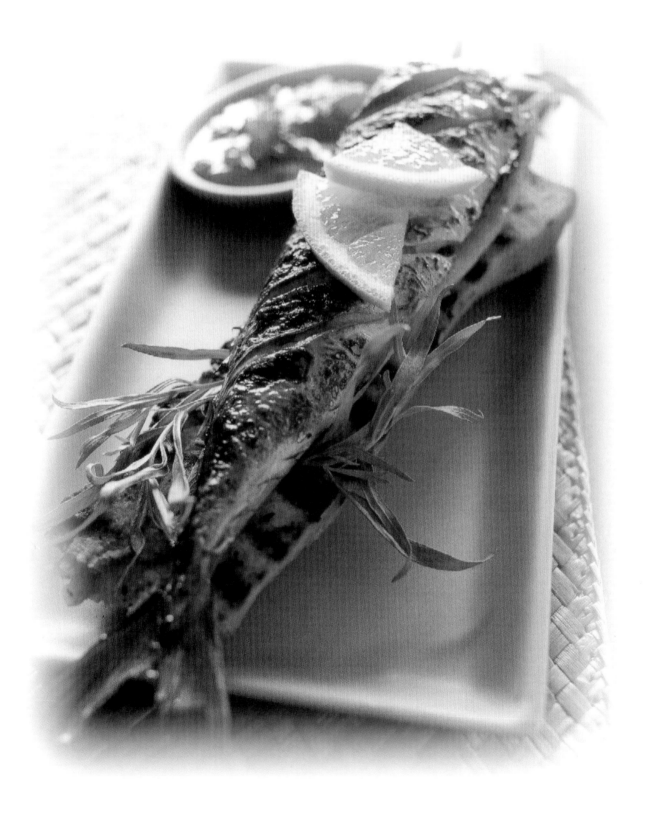

FISH TWISTS WITH LIME SAUCE

SERVES **4**

These colourful fish twists are perfect for a dinner party, or when you want to impress without spending hours in the kitchen. They are also a delightful alternative to crab sticks. Plaice is also a very versatile, low-fat mild fish.

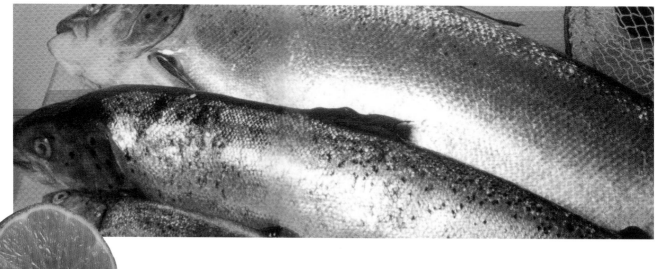

650 g salmon trout fillets, skinned

450 g plaice fillets, skinned

juice and zest of 1 medium lime

1 garlic clove, peeled and crushed

FOR THE SAUCE

8 tbsp plain yoghurt

1 tsp lime juice

1 tsp lemon juice

1 garlic clove, peeled and crushed

2 tbsp fresh parsley, chopped

TO GARNISH

lime wedges and dill

1 Rinse the fillets under running water and pat dry. Cut the salmon trout into 8 strips and the plaice into 4. Trim fish fillets into identical lengths. On a chopping board twist 2 salmon trout fillets around one plaice fillet.

2 Line a steamer tier with greaseproof paper and place the fish twists in the steamer tier with the lime and garlic.

3 Cover with a tight-fitting lid and steam over boiling water for 10 minutes or until the fish is cooked through.

4 After 5 minutes cooking time, begin to make the sauce. Blend the yoghurt, lime juice and lemon juice in a food processor. Stir in the garlic and parsley and transfer the sauce to a mixing bowl.

5 Stand the bowl over a saucepan of hot water while transferring the cooked fish onto warmed plates. Spoon the sauce around the fish, and garnish with lime wedges and dill. Serve immediately.

NUTRITIONAL VALUES

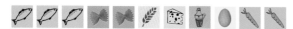

OATY MACKEREL

SERVES **4**

A simple, delicious variation on traditional herrings in oats.

1 Put the oats on a plate and season well. Hold one mackerel by its tail and sprinkle the flesh side with a little lemon juice. Press the fish on the oats, flesh side down and use a spoon to dust more oats over the top of the fish. Press the oats on well, then lay the mackerel on the grill rack. Repeat with the remaining mackerel.

2 Cook the mackerel under a moderately hot grill, allowing about 10 minutes on each side, until the oats are browned and crisp and the fish is cooked through.

3 Serve piping hot, with thinly sliced wholemeal bread.

8 tbsp medium steel-cut oats

freshly ground black pepper

4 small mackerel, gutted with heads off and boned

a little lemon juice

NUTRITIONAL VALUES

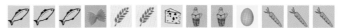

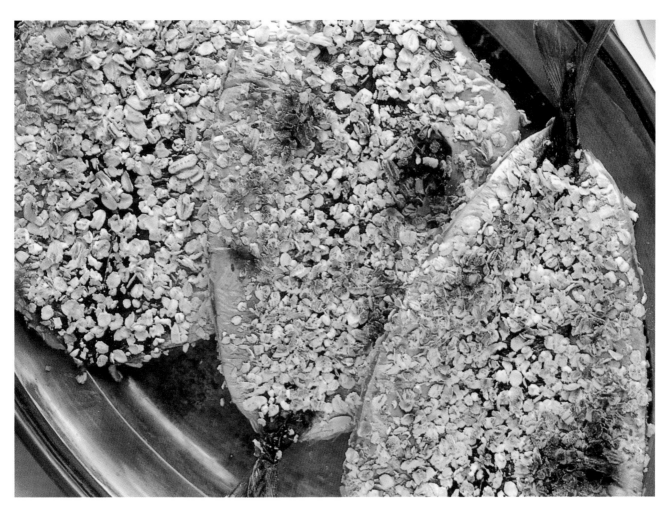

TROUT WITH FLAGEOLET BEAN SALAD

SERVES **2**

This pretty, pale pink and green salad makes a good light meal or appetizer. Serve with plenty of crusty bread to mop up the juices.

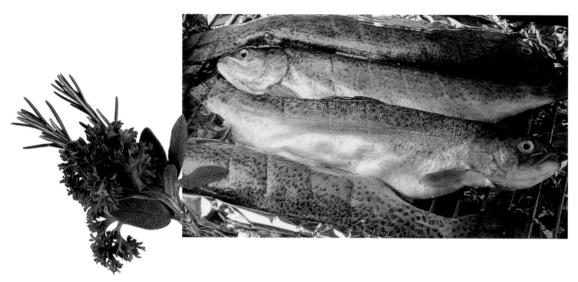

1 trout, weighing about 275 g

2 lemon slices

2 sprigs parsley

400 g can flageolet beans

2 small–medium tomatoes, skinned, seeded, and
   cut into 0.5 cm cubes

1 tbsp chopped chives or parsley

37 g walnuts, broken up and roasted lightly in a dry
   frying pan

freshly ground black pepper

FOR THE VINAIGRETTE

1 tbsp walnut oil

1 tbsp olive oil

1 tbsp white wine vinegar

¹/₂ small garlic clove, minced

1   Preheat the oven to 190°C/gas mark 5.

2   Put the trout on a large piece of oiled foil, insert the lemon slices and parsley sprigs in the cavity, and season inside and out with pepper. Wrap loosely in the foil and bake for 15–20 minutes (to check if the trout is done, insert a knife near the backbone; the flesh should flake but still be moist). Allow to cool. Remove the skin and bones, separate the flesh into chunks, and season well with pepper.

3   Drain the beans, rinse well, and pat dry on paper towels. Put them in a shallow dish with the diced tomatoes.

4   To prepare the vinaigrette, whisk together all the ingredients; season well with pepper and toss about three-quarters of it with the beans.

5   Stir in most of the chives and parsley and most of the trout, saving a few chunks of trout to garnish. Arrange these on top of the salad, then sprinkle over the walnuts and the remaining herbs, drizzle over the remaining dressing, and serve.

NUTRITIONAL VALUES

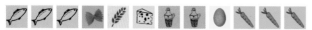

FISH PROVENÇAL

SERVES **4**

When cooking fish in the slow cooker it is best to skin it first. Slip a long sharp knife under the skin at the tail end, then slip it down the length of the fish or, if the fish is firm fleshed, rip the skin off.

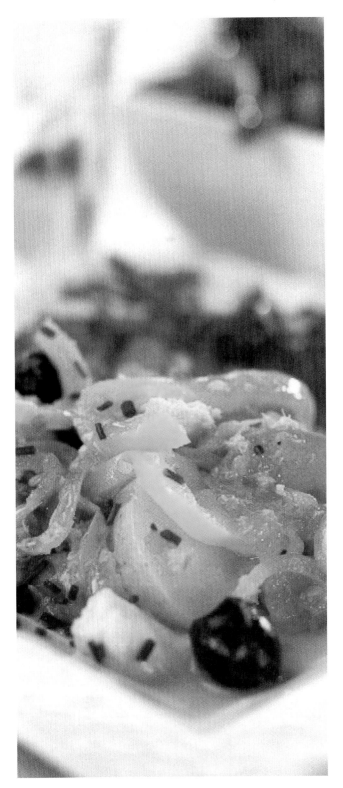

4 cod or other firm white fish fillets, about 550 g

1 onion, peeled and sliced

1 yellow pepper, deseeded and sliced

425 g can artichoke hearts, drained and cut in half

4 firm tomatoes, sliced

2 oz pitted black olives

1 bay leaf

freshly ground black pepper

120 ml medium dry white wine

TO GARNISH

snipped fresh olives

TO SERVE

warm crusty bread or new potatoes and salad

NUTRITIONAL VALUES

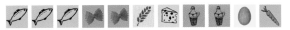

1   Preheat the slow cooker on high. Skin the fish if necessary, cut into bite-sized pieces and place in the cooking pot. Add the remaining ingredients except for the wine and chives. Bring the wine to just below boiling point, pour over the fish, then cover with the lid.

2   Reduce the temperature to low and cook for 3–4 hours. Serve garnished with chives and with either warm crusty bread or new potatoes and salad.

FISH AND VEGETABLE CASSEROLE

SERVES **8–10**

Cod, haddock or monkfish would all be suitable types of fish to use for this dish, which originates from the Greek island of Corfu. The crucial ingredient is the garlic, and plenty of it.

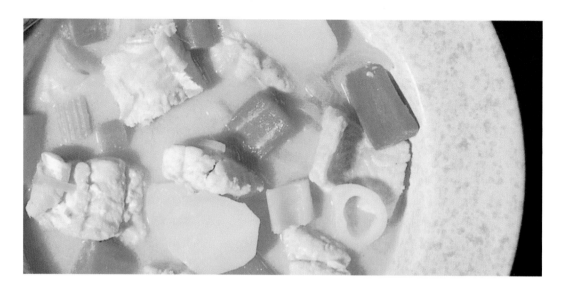

NUTRITIONAL VALUES

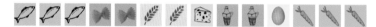

6 tbsp olive oil

1 large onion, sliced

900 g small potatoes, washed and cut into 1 cm
   slices

2 carrots, cut into 2.5 cm chunks

1 celery stick, chopped

salt substitute (see page 15) and freshly ground
   black pepper

6 garlic cloves, crushed

1.2 kg firm white fish fillets, skinned and cut into
   5 cm chunks

60 ml freshly squeezed lemon juice

1 Heat the olive oil in a large, heavy saucepan and sauté the onion for about 3 minutes or until softened and slightly brown.

2 Add the potatoes, carrots and celery, and season with the salt substitute and freshly ground black pepper. Continue to cook for a further 4–5 minutes or until the vegetables begin to soften.

3 Stir in the garlic and pour over enough boiling water to just cover the vegetables. Bring to the boil, cover, and simmer for 10–15 minutes or until the vegetables are almost tender.

4 Gently stir the fish into the casserole, cover, and simmer for 10–15 minutes or until the fish flakes easily. Add a little extra water if necessary. Just before the end of the cooking time, remove the cover and stir in the lemon juice and remaining olive oil.

5 Adjust the seasoning if necessary and serve.

MOROCCAN WHOLE FISH BAKED WITH CUMIN

SERVES **4**

The spicy mixture of cumin, coriander and garlic, all bound up in olive oil, makes a delicious flavouring for fish. It is used here on a whole fish for roasting, but you could also use it on pieces of fish wrapped in baking parchment, then roasted in their own steam and juices, or as a paste for portions of fish to be steamed.

1 whole fish, such as a striped bass or snapper, about 1.5–1.75 kg, cleaned but with head and tail left on

1 tbsp salt substitute (see page 15)

1 lemon, cut into halves (one for juice, and one to cut in wedges for a garnish)

125 g extra virgin olive oil

3 tbsp ground cumin

2 tbsp paprika

25 g chopped fresh coriander

5 garlic cloves, chopped

freshly ground black pepper

1 Preheat the oven to 200°C/gas mark 6. Wash the fish, then cut slashes on its outside skin. Rub half the salt substitute and lemon juice into the cuts and inside the fish. Leave to sit for 15–25 minutes. Rinse with cold water, and dry with a paper towel.

2 Combine the olive oil, cumin, paprika, coriander, garlic and pepper and mix into a paste. Rub the paste over the skin of the fish, inside and out, also inside the slashes.

3 Place the fish on a baking sheet and roast for 30–40 minutes, or until the fish is done; its flesh will feel firm but not hard. Take care not to overcook.

4 Serve hot, accompanied by wedges of lemon, and a cruet of olive oil if desired, for drizzling.

NUTRITIONAL VALUES

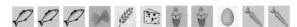

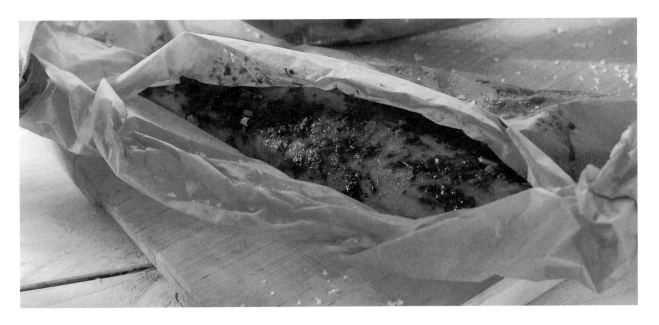

MONKFISH, CAULIFLOWER AND SNOW PEAS

SERVES **4**

This is a very popular dish in Singapore. It can be easily cooked in a microwave and served with a bowl of brown rice.

½ cauliflower

2 tbsp water

330 g snow peas

330 g monkfish pieces (or other
   firm white fish, such as
   grouper)

2 tbsp dry sherry

2 tbsp soy sauce

1 garlic clove, crushed

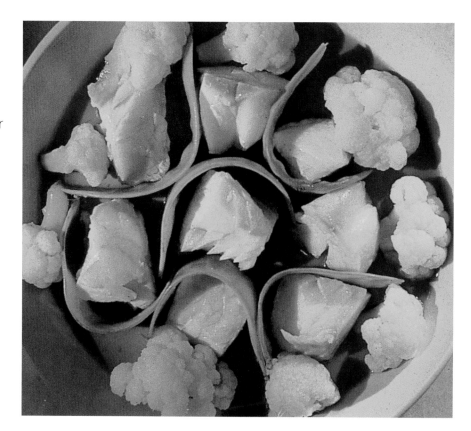

NUTRITIONAL VALUES

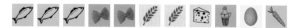

1 Break the cauliflower into florets, discarding tough stems and leaves. Put it in a microwave-safe bowl with the water, cover and cook on full for 3–4 minutes, until you can pierce the stems with the point of a sharp knife. Stir once during cooking.

2 String the snow peas. Put the cauliflower and peas in a microwave-safe bowl with the monkfish.

3 Combine the sherry, soy sauce and garlic. Pour over the vegetables and monkfish, stirring well. Leave for 30 minutes to marinate, stirring occasionally.

4 Cover the bowl with vented plastic wrap and cook on full for 3 minutes, stirring once. Serve immediately.

POACHED MARINATED FISH

SERVES **4**

A very tasty main meal of fish, ideally served with fresh, crusty, granary bread which can also be served in smaller portions as a starter.

1.25 litre water

6 tbsp fresh lime or lemon juice

2 tsp salt substitute (see page 15)

2 x 450 g fish, scaled, cleaned and cut into four steaks about 2.5 cm thick (snapper, sea bream, or mullet)

1 small onion, finely chopped

1 tsp crushed garlic cloves

1 chilli pepper, chopped

2 bay leaves

1/2 tsp dried thyme

2 spring onions, chopped

2 sprigs fresh thyme

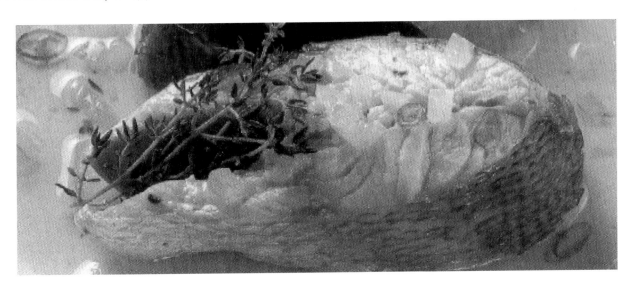

NUTRITIONAL VALUES

1 Put half the water, half the lime or lemon juice, and salt substitute into a large, shallow, glass baking dish. Wash the fish steaks under cold running water, then put them in the baking dish and leave to marinade for about 1 hour.

2 Drain and discard the marinade. Pour the remaining water into a frying pan with the onion, garlic, hot pepper, bay leaves and thyme. Bring to the boil over high heat, then lower the heat and simmer for 5 minutes.

3 Add the fish steaks to the pan and bring back to the boil. Reduce the heat to the lowest setting, cover the pan, and simmer for 10 minutes, or until the fish flakes easily when tested with the tip of a knife.

4 Transfer the fish to a warmed serving dish. Add the remaining lime or lemon juice to the cooking liquid, then pour this over the fish. Taste to check the seasoning, then serve at once, garnished with fresh thyme and chopped spring onion. Serve with fresh granary bread.

GRILLED TUNA WITH ORANGE, THYME AND GARLIC

SERVES **6**

The flavours of orange and tuna complement each other wonderfully well. In this recipe thin slices of garlic are pushed into the tuna steaks, creating an intensely garlicky dish.

NUTRITIONAL VALUES

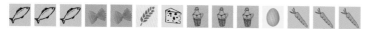

juice of 1 large orange

3 plump garlic cloves, very thinly sliced

2 tbsp fresh thyme leaves

1 tbsp finely grated orange rind

ground black pepper

6 tuna steaks, about 2.5 cm thick.

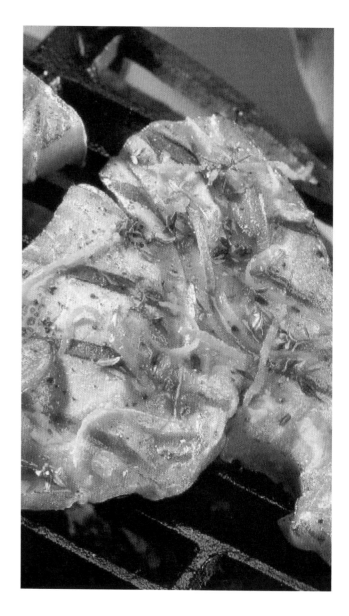

1   Put the orange juice, thyme, orange rind and seasoning into a shallow non-metallic dish, large enough to hold the tuna in a single layer. Mix well, then add the tuna steaks, turning them until evenly coated. Push some of the garlic slices between the flakes of tuna.

2   Cover and leave to marinate in the refrigerator for 30 minutes–1 hour, turning the tuna once or twice during this time.

3   Lift the fish out of its marinade and cook over medium–high heat for about 4–5 minutes on each side or until very nearly cooked through. (Tuna becomes rather dry if overcooked, so stop cooking when it is still slightly translucent at the centre.)

SALMON AND BROCCOLI PENNE

SERVES **4**

Steaming this delicious pasta sauce retains all of the wonderful colours, textures and flavours of the fish and broccoli for a perfect supper dish. Use trout fillets in place of salmon if preferred.

350 g dry penne

250 g broccoli florets

1/2 tbsp olive oil

1 tsp garlic wine vinegar

2 garlic cloves, peeled and crushed

juice and zest of 1 medium orange

350 g salmon fillet, skinned and cut
  into cubes

6 tbsp dry white wine

150 ml low-fat fromage frais

2 tbsp fresh dill, chopped

2 tbsp freshly grated Parmesan
  cheese

freshly ground black pepper

TO GARNISH

orange wedges and dill

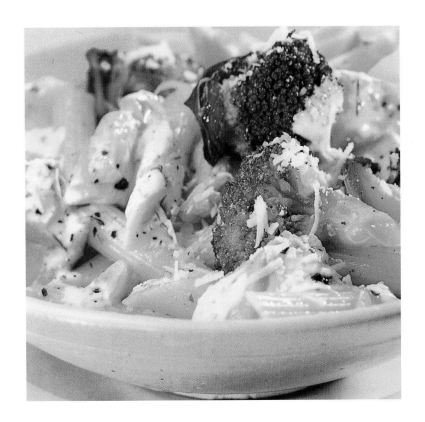

NUTRITIONAL VALUES

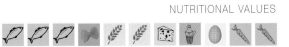

1   Half fill the steamer base with water and bring to the boil. Add the pasta and season with a little salt (add it later for pasta to be firm to the bite).

2   Place the broccoli in a greaseproof paper-lined steamer tier. Mix the oil, vinegar, garlic and orange juice and rind together and pour over the broccoli. Rinse the salmon under running water and pat dry. Add the salmon to the pan and cover with a tight-fitting lid.

3   Set on top of the pasta in boiling water for 10 minutes or until the pasta and fish are cooked through.

4   Meanwhile, heat the wine, low-fat fromage frais, dill and Parmesan in a saucepan to just below boiling point. Season to taste.

5   Drain the pasta and transfer to a warmed serving dish. Spoon the fish and broccoli on top and spoon the sauce over. Garnish, and serve immediately.

MACKEREL WITH SPICY TOMATO JAM

SERVES **4**

Mackerel is a very oily, medium-firm fish that contains a high level of vitamin A, so this comforting dish is very good for you. Mackerel is at its best around spring and summer.

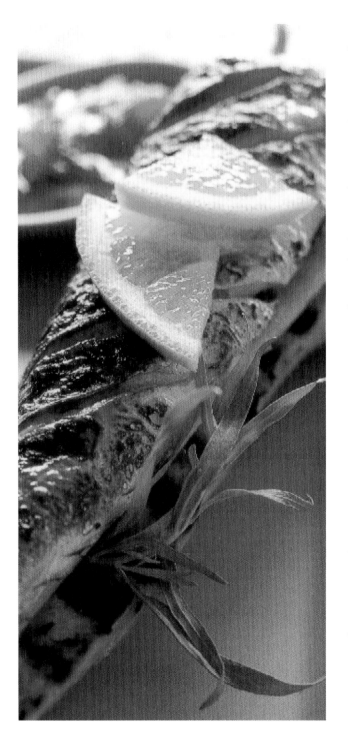

450 g tomatoes, skinned, deseeded and chopped

1 medium Spanish onion, diced

125 ml apple jelly

50 ml cider vinegar

1 tbsp chopped tarragon

$^{1}/_{2}$–1 tsp crushed red chilli pepper

four 225 g mackerel fillets, cleaned, with heads removed but with the skin left on

olive oil

freshly ground black pepper to taste

TO GARNISH

sprigs of tarragon and orange slices

1 Combine the tomato, onion, jelly, vinegar, tarragon and red chilli pepper in a medium saucepan. Bring to the boil over a medium–high heat. Reduce the heat to medium–low and cook, stirring frequently, 35–45 minutes or until thick. Cool the jam to room temperature.

2 Season the mackerel with pepper and brush the skin with olive oil. Grill, skin side down, covered, over medium–high heat, 5 minutes on each side. Do not turn the fish or overcook it.

3 To serve, top each fillet with 2 tablespoons of tomato jam and season to taste. Garnish with tarragon and orange slices.

NUTRITIONAL VALUES

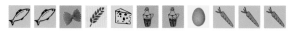

TROUT WITH WILD RICE STUFFING

SERVES **4**

Wild rice makes excellent stuffing. It goes well with game birds, such as pheasant and duck, or with fish. It is best not to mix the stuffing with egg when using fish, as a crumbly stuffing seems to go better with the flaky fish texture.

4 trout, brown or rainbow

STUFFING

1 small onion, finely chopped

1 stick celery, finely sliced

1 tbsp oil

1/2 small green pepper, finely chopped

1 garlic clove, crushed

150 g cooked wild rice (about 50 g raw)

1 tbsp freshly chopped dill or parsley

1 lemon, grated rind and juice

freshly ground black pepper

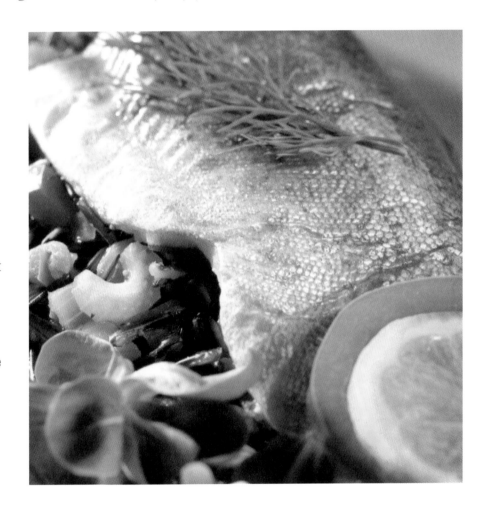

1 Preheat an oven to 200°C/gas mark 6. Lightly oil a suitable ovenproof dish.

2 Cook the onion and celery in the oil until softened but not browned. Add the pepper and continue cooking until all the vegetables are soft. Remove the pan from the heat and stir in the garlic and cooked rice. Add the herbs, lemon rind and juice, then season to taste with the freshly ground black pepper.

3 Clean the trout, removing the heads if preferred. Season the cavities lightly and fill with the stuffing. Arrange the fish in the prepared dish and cover with foil. Bake for 15–20 minutes, according to the size of the fish, until just cooked. Serve immediately while still hot.

NUTRITIONAL VALUES

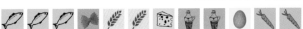

COUSCOUS-STUFFED TOMATOES WITH SMOKED TOFU AND TUNA

SERVES **6**

Choose large, even-sized beefsteak tomatoes that are ripe but still firm for this delicious and healthy dish.

6 large beefsteak tomatoes

1 tbsp olive oil

1 garlic clove, peeled and crushed

3 spring onions, chopped

150 g couscous

a few saffron threads

250 ml fish stock

1 tbsp tomato purée

150 g smoked tofu, finely diced

100 g tin of tuna in brine, drained and flaked

freshly ground black pepper

NUTRITIONAL VALUES

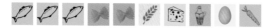

1 Cut the tops off the tomatoes and scoop out the pulp and seeds with a teaspoon, taking care not to split the skins. Sieve the pulp and reserve, discarding the seeds. Stand the tomatoes upside down on a plate to drain.

2 Heat the oil in a frying pan and sauté the garlic and scallions until soft. Add the couscous, saffron and all but 2 tablespoons of the stock. Mix the tomato paste with the sieved pulp and stir in. Cover the pan and simmer for 10–15 minutes until the couscous has swollen and absorbed the liquid, stirring occasionally.

3 Remove from the heat, stir in the smoked tofu and tuna, and season with pepper. Preheat the oven to 180°C/gas mark 4.

4 Spoon the filling into the tomato shells, packing down firmly. Stand the tomatoes in a shallow baking pan and replace the tops. Spoon over the reserved stock and bake uncovered for 15–20 minutes until the tomatoes are tender but not falling apart. Serve hot.

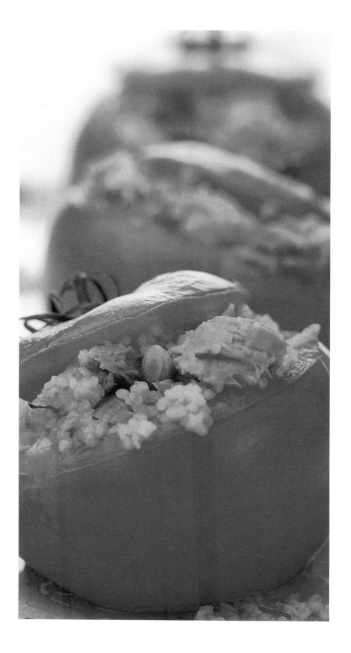

TABBOULEH WITH TOFU, RAISINS AND PINENUTS

SERVES **4**

An aromatic Middle Eastern salad made with bulgur wheat, fragrant fresh parsley and mint. Make ahead of time and leave for several hours or overnight before serving, to allow the flavours to develop.

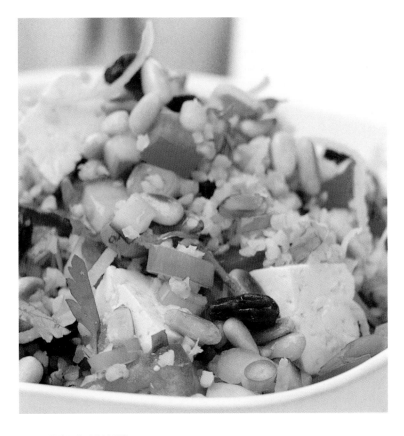

125 g bulgur wheat

7 tbsp extra virgin olive oil

50 g pinenuts

grated rind and juice of 1 lemon

2 garlic cloves, peeled and crushed

1 small cucumber

2 tomatoes

4 tbsp raisins

8 spring onions, finely chopped

4 tbsp chopped fresh flat-leaved parsley

2 tbsp chopped fresh mint

250 g firm tofu, cubed

pepper

NUTRITIONAL VALUES

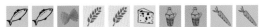

1 Put the bulgur wheat in a large bowl, cover with cold water, and leave to soak for at least 30 minutes. Heat 1 tablespoon of the olive oil in a small frying pan and stir-fry the pinenuts briefly until golden. Drain on a plate lined with kitchen paper.

2 Mix together the remaining olive oil with the lemon juice and garlic. Dice the cucumber and chop the tomatoes into small pieces.

3 Drain the bulgur wheat in a strainer, shaking out as much excess water as possible. Place in a bowl and add the cucumber, tomatoes, raisins, spring onions, parsley, mint and tofu.

4 Pour the oil and lemon dressing over the mixture, and toss well. Add seasoning to taste. Cover the bowl and leave in a cool place for several hours or overnight. Sprinkle with the pinenuts and grated lemon rind when ready to serve.

POTATO-TOPPED VEGETABLE PIE

SERVES **4**

Cook the potatoes whole in their skins to retain maximum nutrients; once cooked they can be easily peeled and mashed. This dish can be prepared the previous day if necessary.

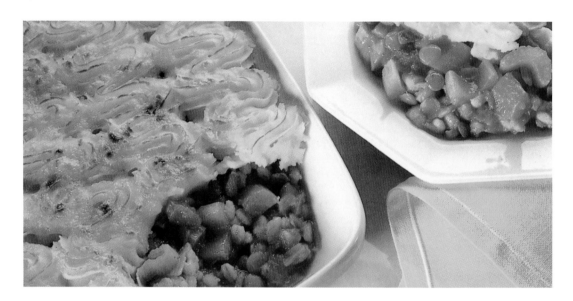

75 g green lentils, washed and drained

50 g pot barley, washed and drained

1 medium onion, chopped

400 g can chopped tomatoes

175 g cauliflower florets

2 celery stalks, sliced

1 leek, thickly sliced

1 turnip, thinly sliced

2 carrots, diced

2 tsp mixed dry herbs

750 g potatoes, scrubbed

3 tbsp semi-skimmed milk

pepper

25 g low-fat medium-hard cheese, grated

1 Set the oven to 200°C/gas mark 6. Place the lentils, barley, onion, tomatoes (with juice), cauliflower, celery, leek, turnip, carrots and herbs in a large saucepan and add 300 ml water. Bring to the boil, cover and simmer for 40–45 minutes or until the lentils, barley and vegetables are just tender.

2 Cook the potatoes in boiling water for about 20 minutes, or until they are soft. Drain, peel and mash them with the milk and season to taste.

3 Place the lentil mixture into a pie dish and pipe or fork the mashed potato on top to cover. Sprinkle on the cheese and bake the pie in the oven for 30–35 minutes, until it is evenly light brown.

4 Serve hot. A tomato and herb salad makes a good accompaniment.

NUTRITIONAL VALUES

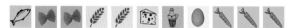

SPICED MINCED CHICKEN

SERVES **6**

One of the special characteristics of the northeastern Thai version of this dish is the addition of uncooked sticky rice, which is first roasted (either in an oven or in a dry wok) until golden and then pounded in a mortar. It adds a slightly nutty flavour and gives the dish more body.

450 g finely minced chicken

25 g shallots, sliced

10 g coriander leaves

4 tbsp sticky rice, dry-fried for 8–10 minutes until brown and finely pounded

4 tbsp lemon juice, or to taste

3 tbsp fish sauce, or to taste

1 tbsp chopped dried red chilli, or to taste

TO GARNISH

fresh mint leaves

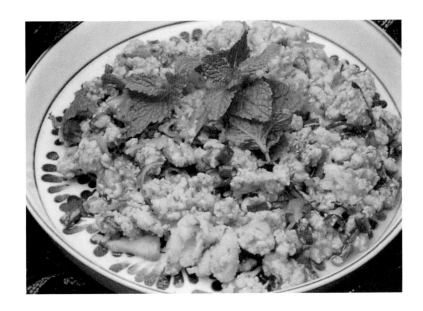

1 Cook the chicken in a non-stick pan over low heat for 10 minutes – do not add water or oil. When cooked, transfer to a bowl and mix in well all the remaining ingredients except the mint.

2 Check the seasoning, and add more lemon juice, fish sauce or chilli if necessary. Sprinkle the mint over the top to garnish.

3 Serve accompanied by raw cabbage leaves, spring onions and raw green beans.

NUTRITIONAL VALUES

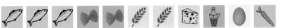

CHICKEN, MUSHROOM AND SPINACH LASAGNE

SERVES **6**

A tasty lasagne, accompanied with a crisp salad and crusty brown bread makes for easy and informal entertaining. Prepare the lasagne in advance and chill until you are ready to cook it.

NUTRITIONAL VALUES

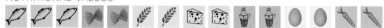

CHICKEN AND NUTMEG SAUCE

4 tbsp olive oil

1 small onion, finely chopped

500 g uncooked chicken meat, cut into 1.5 cm
  cubes

125 g plain flour

900 ml semi-skimmed milk

¹/₂ tsp freshly grated nutmeg

freshly ground black pepper

MUSHROOM AND SPINACH MIXTURE

1 tbsp olive oil

1 onion, finely chopped

3 garlic cloves, crushed

375 g flat mushrooms, finely chopped

375 g fresh spinach, washed

freshly ground black pepper

300–375 g green pre-cooked lasagne
  (approx. 12 sheets)

50 g Parmesan cheese, freshly grated

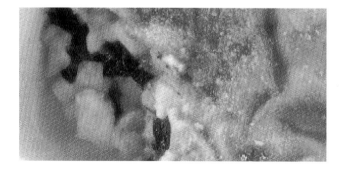

1 To make the chicken sauce, heat 1 tablespoon of the oil in a pan and cook the onion gently until softened. Add the diced chicken and stir-fry until the chicken is firm and cooked through.

2 In another saucepan, heat the remaining oil. Add the flour and cook, stirring, for one minute. Remove from the heat and slowly blend in the milk, beating to a smooth sauce between each addition. Return to the heat and bring to the boil and cook for one minute. Season with the nutmeg and pepper.

3 Put a third of the sauce into a bowl and reserve. Add the chicken and onion mixture to the remaining sauce. Place a layer of damp greaseproof paper on the surface of both sauces to prevent a skin forming.

4 For the mushroom and spinach mixture, heat the oil and cook the onion and garlic gently until softened. Add the mushrooms and cook gently for 10 minutes or until any liquid has evaporated.

5 Cook the spinach briefly in a large covered saucepan until it has wilted and reduced in volume. No need to add any water. Drain, squeeze out any excess liquid and then chop finely. Add to the mushroom mixture and season to taste.

6 Lightly oil a deep rectangular ovenproof dish approx. 30 x 18 cm. Line the bottom and sides of the dish with some of the pasta and then a thin layer with half the chicken sauce, pasta, spinach and mushroom sauce, more pasta, the remaining chicken sauce, pasta and the plain sauce.

7 Sprinkle with the grated Parmesan and cook for 45–50 minutes or until bubbling and golden brown on top.

TOMATO AND CHICKEN CASSEROLE

SERVES **4 – 6**

A warming, tasty and colourful chicken dish, that should ideally be served with new potatoes or jacket potatoes.

50 ml olive oil

1.5 kg prepared chicken, cut into portions

flour, for dredging

2 large red onions, sliced

2 x 400 g cans chopped tomatoes

3 garlic cloves, crushed

freshly ground black pepper, to taste

75 g boiling water

2 tbsp red wine vinegar

TO GARNISH

chopped fresh parsley

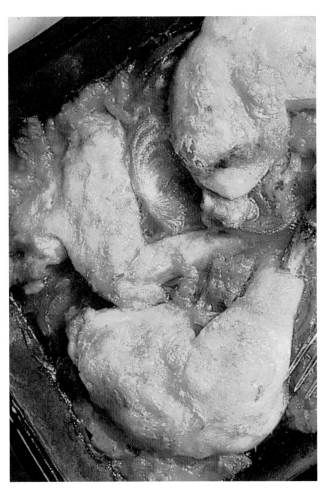

1 Preheat the oven to 190°C/gas mark 5. Heat the oil in a large, flameproof casserole. Place the chicken portions on a chopping board and dredge all over with flour. Place in casserole and cook for about 5 minutes, or until evenly browned, turning the portions as they cook. Using a slotted spoon, transfer the chicken portions to a plate and set aside.

2 Add the onion to the casserole and cook for 3 minutes, or until softened. Return the chicken to the casserole, add the chopped tomatoes and garlic and season with the freshly ground black pepper. Add the boiling water, cover, and cook in the oven for 45–55 minutes or until the chicken is tender and the sauce has thickened.

3 In the last 5 minutes of cooking time, stir in the red wine vinegar and a little extra boiling water if necessary. Serve sprinkled with chopped fresh parsley.

NUTRITIONAL VALUES

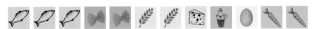

MEXICAN RICE CHICKEN

SERVES **6**

This recipe adds chicken to authentic spicy Mexican or Spanish rice.

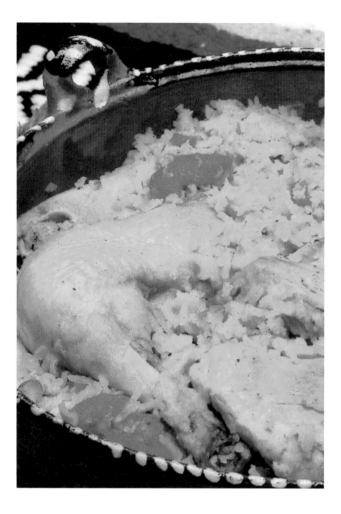

1.5–1.75 g chicken

2 medium onions, finely chopped

2 garlic cloves, chopped

2 serrano chillies, chopped

450 g tomatoes, peeled and de-seeded, or canned
   tomatoes

50 ml olive oil

450 g long grain rice

$^1/_4$ tsp whole cumin seed

$^1/_4$ tsp saffron

900 ml chicken stock

pepper

200 g frozen peas

1 Cut the chicken into serving pieces. Fry until golden; drain and set aside. In the same oil, fry the chopped or sliced onion together with the garlic. Drain, and add to the chicken, together with the tomatoes, stock and spices. Bring to the boil; simmer for about half an hour.

2 Meanwhile, still in the same oil – adding a little more if necessary – fry the rice until it is golden, stirring frequently. Add the rice to the chicken; mix well; bring back to the boil, stirring frequently.

3 When the rice has absorbed all the visible liquid (10–20 minutes), add the peas; stir briefly; then cover tightly and simmer over a very low heat for another 20 minutes or so.

NUTRITIONAL VALUES

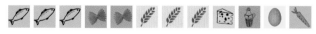

CARIBBEAN CHICKEN CASSEROLE

SERVES **6**

This is a lovely summer casserole with a distinctive flavour that makes you think of the hot Caribbean sunshine.

1.5 kg chicken, cut into 5 cm pieces

1 tsp freshly ground black pepper

2 garlic cloves

¼ tsp vinegar

1 bayleaf

2 tbsp olive oil

1 medium tomato, chopped

2 celery sticks, chopped

2 carrots, diced

¼ cabbage, shredded

4 potatoes, chopped

175 g green beans, cleaned

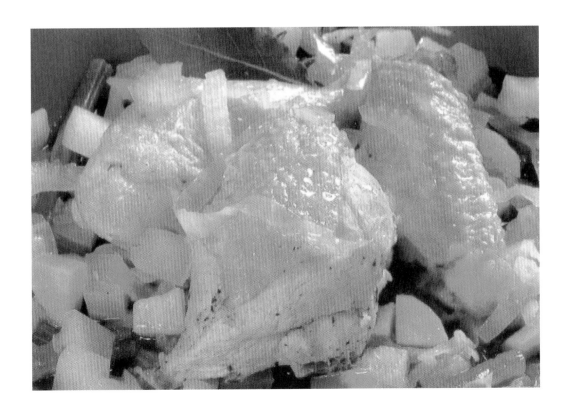

1   Wash the chicken. Marinate the pieces in a bowl with the pepper, garlic, thyme, bayleaf and vinegar for 5 hours.

2   Heat the oil in a large saucepan, then add the tomatoes and chicken pieces. Cover with cold water, bring it to the boil, then lower and heat and simmer, covered, for 30 minutes or until the chicken is almost cooked and the liquid has reduced.

3   Add the onion and the other vegetables, and cook until they are tender but crisp.

4   Serve immediately with fresh bread or boiled rice and hot pepper sauce.

NUTRITIONAL VALUES

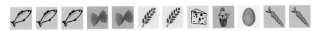

TURKEY IN CHOCOLATE SAUCE

SERVES **4**

To many the idea of adding chocolate to a savoury dish may seem a little strange but Mexican chocolate is bitter, not at all like the chocolate we know. Use the darkest unsweetened chocolate you can find. Chicken is everyday fare in Mexico, while turkey is kept for festivals and special occasions. If the dried chillies are unavailable, use the darkest chilli powder you can find.

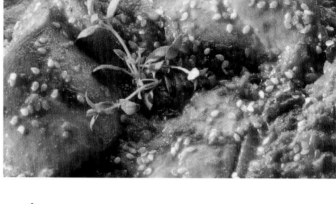

3 dried ancho chillies

3 dried pasilla chillies

3 dried mulato chillies

1 onion, sliced

2 garlic cloves, crushed

25 g sesame seeds, toasted

25 g blanched almonds, cut into slivers and
    toasted

1 tsp ground coriander

$\frac{1}{2}$ tsp freshly ground black pepper

few cloves

3–4 tbsp olive oil

300 ml chicken stock

450 g tomatoes, peeled, deseeded and chopped

2 tsp ground cinnamon

50 g raisins

50 g pumpkin seeds, toasted

50 g dark chocolate, melted

1 tbsp red wine vinegar

8 turkey thigh portions or 4 boneless chicken
    breasts

1 Roast the dried chillies and rehydrate then put into a food processor or pestle and mortar with the onion, garlic, sesame seeds, almonds, coriander, black pepper and cloves. Grind to form a paste.

2 Heat 2 tablespoons of the oil in a heavy-based pan and gently sauté the paste for 5 minutes, stirring frequently.

3 Add 150 ml of the stock, the tomatoes, cinnamon, raisins and pumpkin seeds. Bring to the boil, then reduce the heat and simmer for 15 minutes, or until a thick consistency is reached. Stir in the melted chocolate and vinegar, mixing together well, cover and keep warm and reserve.

4 Meanwhile, heat the remaining oil in a frying pan and seal the turkey thighs or chicken breasts on all sides. Drain off the oil and add the remaining stock. Bring to the boil, then reduce the heat and simmer for 15 minutes, or until tender and drain off any liquor.

5 Pour the sauce over the turkey or chicken and reheat gently. Serve garnished with roasted sesame seeds and fresh herbs.

TO GARNISH

extra sesame seeds, toasted, and fresh herbs

NUTRITIONAL VALUES

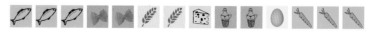

TURKEY TAGINE

SERVES **4**

This recipe takes its inspiration from Morocco. It is cooked in a slow cooker and served with couscous.

450 g diced turkey meat

2 tbsp flour

freshly ground black pepper

2 tbsp olive oil

1 medium onion, peeled and sliced into wedges

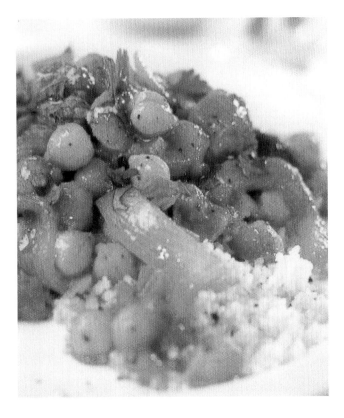

3–4 garlic cloves, peeled and sliced

1 tsp ground cumin

1 tsp ground coriander

1 cinnamon stick, lightly bashed

large pinch of saffron

2 large carrots, peeled and sliced

300 ml turkey or chicken stock

75 g chopped dried apricots

3 tomatoes, chopped

400 g can chickpeas, drained

TO GARNISH

1 tbsp chopped fresh coriander

TO SERVE

steamed couscous and bread or other green salad

NUTRITIONAL VALUES

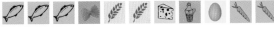

1 Preheat the slow cooker on high. Trim and discard any sinew or fat from the meat, then toss in the flour seasoned with salt and pepper. Heat 1 tablespoon of the oil in a pan and gently sauté the onion and garlic for 3 minutes. With a slotted spoon, transfer to the cooking pot.

2 Add the remaining oil to the pan and sear the turkey meat on all sides. Sprinkle in the ground spices with the cinnamon stick and saffron, add the carrots and cook, stirring frequently, for 3 minutes. Add the stock, stirring throughout. Bring to the boil, add the apricots and tomatoes, then pour over the onions in the cooking pot and mix lightly.

3 Cover the cooking pot with the lid and cook for 2 hours. Add the drained chick peas and continue to cook for another 1–3 hours. Remove the cinnamon stick, stir in the chopped coriander and serve with the freshly prepared couscous and bread or a green salad.

RABBIT STEW WITH LEEKS AND WILD MUSHROOMS

SERVES **4**

Wild mushrooms give this stew a heavenly accent. It is not a difficult dish. Start a day ahead by marinating the rabbit pieces, then use the marinade as part of the stewing liquid. The stew forms an excellent gravy.

1.5 kg rabbit, cut into 8 serving pieces

60 ml olive oil

120 ml dry white wine

2 sprigs fresh tarragon, bruised to release flavour

1 bay leaf

2 garlic cloves, finely chopped

2 carrots, peeled and sliced

2 leeks, white part only, thinly sliced

dash of freshly ground black pepper

60–120 g flour

475 ml chicken stock

2 tbsp olive oil

225 g wild mushrooms, any combination, quartered

TO SERVE

serve with hot noodles or cooked rice

NUTRITIONAL VALUES

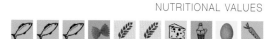

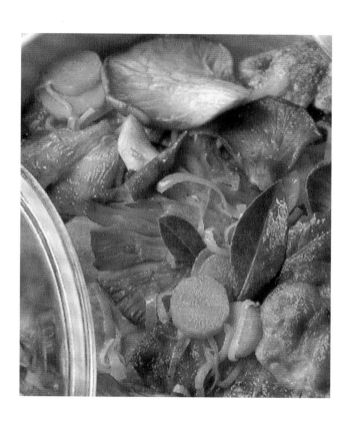

1 In a glass or other non-reactive dish, make the marinade. Combine the olive oil, wine, tarragon, bay leaf, garlic, carrots, 1 leek and ground pepper. Marinate the rabbit for 24 hours in the refrigerator, turning and basting several times.

2 Remove the rabbit and vegetables from the marinade, and discard the bay leaf. Save the marinade. Finely chop the tarragon. Pat the rabbit pieces dry and dredge in flour.

3 In a dutch oven or large pot, heat 2 tablespoons olive oil. Brown the rabbit pieces on all sides, then remove. Sauté the vegetables from the marinade, along with 1 fresh chopped leek. Add the tarragon, rabbit pieces, wine and stock to the pot and bring to the boil. Reduce the heat and simmer for 30 minutes, uncovered. Skim fat from surface.

4 In a small frying pan, add 2 tablespoons olive oil. Sauté the mushrooms for about 7 minutes. Add the mushrooms to the stew, and continue cooking until the rabbit is tender, about 30 minutes longer. Serve the stew over hot noodles or rice.

HARE AND PRUNE CASSEROLE

SERVES **4**

Hare is a notably low-fat meat, and one which fits well into a healthy regime. In this recipe the pieces of lean game meat have been tenderized, first in a spicy marinade and then again by long, slow cooking.

1.5 kg hare joints, washed and dried

6 tbsp wholewheat flour

pepper

1 tbsp dried oregano

3 tbsp olive oil

225 g button onions
   or shallots, peeled
   and left whole

300 ml meat stock

600 ml brown ale

2 tsp wholegrain
   mustard

1 tbsp red wine
   vinegar

1 bouquet garni

225 g no-soak prunes

1 tbsp cornflour

2 tbsp water

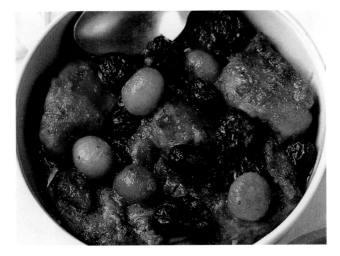

MARINADE

150 ml cider vinegar

150 ml water

1 medium onion, sliced

2 bay leaves

8 peppercorns, lightly
   crushed

8 juniper berries, lightly
   crushed

TO GARNISH

2 Tbsp chopped parsley

NUTRITIONAL VALUES

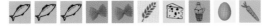

1   Mix together the marinade ingredients in a large bowl. Add the hare joints and spoon the marinade over them. Cover and set aside for several hours, turning once or twice if convenient.

2   Lift out the hare pieces and discard the marinade. Dry the hare joints on kitchen paper. Mix together the flour, pepper and dried oregano and toss the meat in it so that the joints are well coated on all sides. Shake off any excess flour.

3   Heat the oil in a large, heavy-based flameproof casserole or saucepan and brown the onions over medium heat for about 5 minutes, stirring them occasionally. Lift them out with a draining spoon, set aside, then brown the hare joints on all sides. Return the onions to the dish or pan, pour on the stock and beer and stir in the mustard and vinegar. Add the bouquet garni and stir well.

Bring to simmering point, cover and simmer over low heat for 1½ hours, stirring from time to time.

4   Stir in the prunes and continue cooking for 20 minutes, or until the hare is tender. Blend the cornflour to a smooth paste with the water. Set aside.

5   Lift out the hare joints, onions and prunes with a draining spoon, transfer them to a heated serving dish and keep them warm. Discard the bouquet garni.

6   Mix a little of the hot stock with the cornflour paste, then stir it into the pan. Stir over a low heat until the sauce has thickened. Taste and adjust the seasoning if necessary. Pour the sauce over the hare, and sprinkle in the parsley to serve.

GRILLED VENISON STEAKS

SERVES **4**

People often make the mistake of overcooking venison and other game. At the most, it should be cooked to medium, or better yet, medium-rare.

125 ml Italian salad dressing

125 ml soy sauce

2 tbsp spicy mustard

1 tbsp Worcestershire sauce

2 garlic cloves, crushed

freshly ground black pepper

2 venison steaks, 1 cm thick

1 Combine all the marinade ingredients and blend well. Place the steaks and the marinade in a resealable plastic bag, seal and turn to coat. Marinate in the refrigerator for 2–4 hours.

2 Grill the venison over high heat for 3–4 minutes per side, just enough to leave some pink in the middle.

NUTRITIONAL VALUES

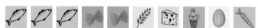

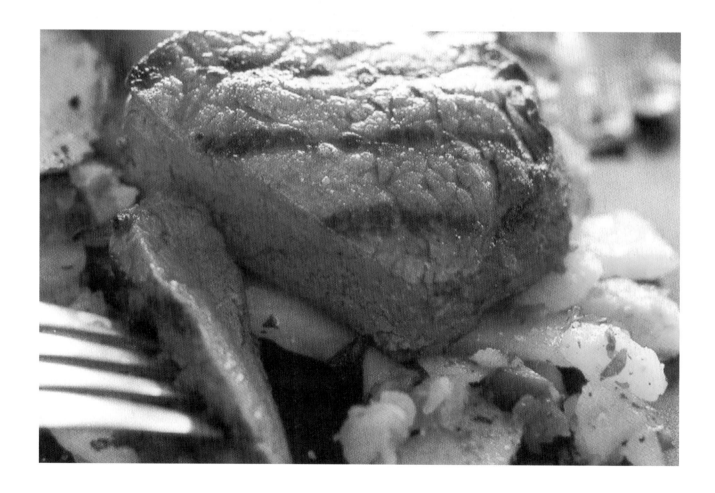

HAYES' VENISON AND BLACK BEAN CHILLI

SERVES **4 – 6**

This chilli dish goes well with Mexican cornbread. If you prefare, beef can be used as a substitute for the venison.

2–3 tbsp olive oil

2–4 garlic cloves, minced

450 g venison tenderloin, cut in thin strips

1 tbsp powdered beef stock cube

black pepper, ground cayenne, ground cumin, crushed red pepper, to taste

1 large white onion, chopped

1 large green pepper, chopped

2–4 fresh chillies, preferably serrano or Thai, chopped

450 g can black beans, undrained

2 x 400 g cans whole tomatoes, undrained

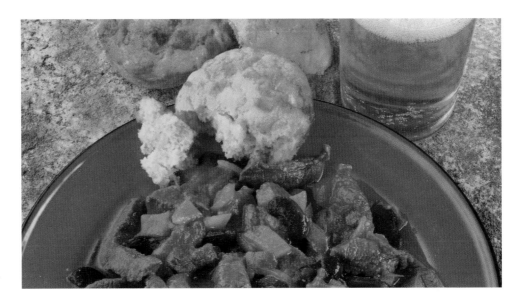

NUTRITIONAL VALUES

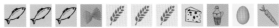

1   Heat the olive oil in a deep iron frying pan and sauté the garlic over medium–high heat until it begins to brown. Add the venison and mix well to distribute the garlic. Stir frequently, cooking until all sides are brown. Add the beef stock. Add the spices to taste – don't be shy – and then stir in the chopped vegetables. Stir until coated with oil and beginning to soften.

2   Stir the undrained beans and tomatoes into the mixture and bring to a rigorous boil. Stir frequently and boil over medium to medium-low heat and cover the pan. Simmer for 45–60 minutes, or until meat is tender and sauce is thick. If possible, cook for several hours, or even a day, before needed. The chilli gets better as it gets older.

LAMB WITH LENTILS AND PRUNES

SERVES **4**

This casserole has many of the clasic flavours of southwest France: plump, moist prunes, green lentils and fresh thyme. The lentils and prunes make it a filling dish and mean that much less meat is required per person than in a more traditional casserole.

2 tbsp olive oil

4 lamb chops or leg steaks, or 450 g lamb fillet, cut
    into 4 pieces

1 large onion, sliced

3 sticks celery, sliced

2 large carrots, sliced

2 plump garlic cloves, finely sliced

1 tbsp fine wholewheat flour

450 ml well-flavoured vegetable or lamb stock

200 g prunes

100 g green lentils

6 juniper berries, lightly crushed

4–5 sprigs fresh thyme

freshly ground black pepper

NUTRITIONAL VALUES

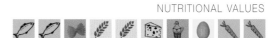

1   Preheat the oven to 160°C/gas mark 3.

2   Heat the oil in a flameproof casserole dish and brown the lamb on all sides. Remove the meat with a slotted spoon and set aside until needed.

3   Add the onion to the casserole and cook slowly until softened but not browned, then add the celery, carrot and garlic and continue cooking for a further 2-3 minutes.

4   Stir the flour into the vegetables and cook for 1-2 minutes, then gradually add the stock, stirring to scrape up any sediment from the bottom of the pan. Bring to the boil; add the prunes and lentils and simmer for 2–3 minutes. Return the lamb to the casserole and add the remaining seasonings.

5   Cover, then cook in the preheated oven for $1\frac{1}{2}$–2 hours. Season to taste before serving the lamb on a bed of the vegetables with the sauce spooned over.

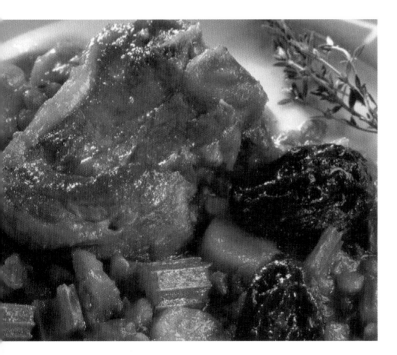

LAMB CASSEROLE

SERVES **6**

A wholesome and warming dish using new or baby potatoes. You can use large potatoes as well, but they work best if you carve them a little into large olive shapes. Especially good on a cold and wintry day!

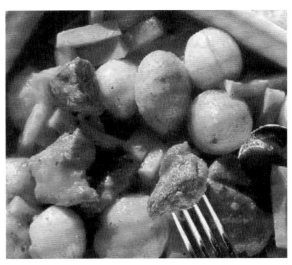

1 boned shoulder of lamb, weighing about 1 kg

4 tbsp olive oil

4 tbsp flour

3 garlic cloves

2 tbsp dried mixed herbs – basil, marjoram, rosemary, oregano or chervil

2 tbsp tomato purée

24 button onions

225 g carrots

450 g new (baby) potatoes

pepper to taste

1 Preheat the oven. Trim the excess fat from the meat and cut into 5 cm cubes.

2 Heat the oil over a medium heat and brown the lamb pieces well.

3 Pour off most of the fat and sprinkle with the flour; cook until it is golden.

4 Crush and stir in the garlic; sauté briefly.

5 Add water to cover the meat, the herbs and the tomato purée, and bring to the boil.

6 Cover the casserole and braise in a warm oven for 1 hour.

7 Meanwhile, peel the onions and cut the carrots into batons. After the hour is up, add them to the casserole.

8 Cook the casserole slowly for a further 45 minutes.

9 Add the little potatoes and continue cooking everything together until the potatoes are tender. If necessary, skim the cooking liquor, season and serve.

NUTRITIONAL VALUES

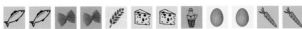

LAMB FILLET WITH PLUM SAUCE

SERVES **4**

This recipe is so simple to prepare and it is absolutely delicious. It will certainly become an all-time favourite, and is ideally suited to cooking in a slow cooker.

2 whole lamb fillets, about 675 g

2 tbsp olive oil

2 tbsp Thai plum sauce

1 tbsp light soy sauce

1 tbsp balsamic vinegar

250 ml orange juice

1 tbsp cornflour

TO GARNISH

flat-leaf parsley and fresh diced plums

TO SERVE

cooked noodles and salad

NUTRITIONAL VALUES

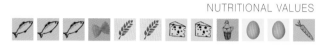

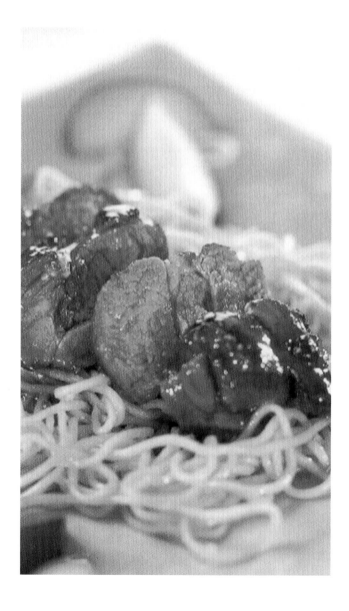

1   Preheat the slow cooker on high. Trim the lamb fillets, heat the olive oil in a large frying pan and sear the fillets on all sides; remove from the pan and reserve.

2   Blend the Thai plum sauce with the soy sauce and vinegar and heat gently. Brush over the top of each fillet, then place the fillets in the cooking pot. Pour over the orange juice, then spoon over any remaining plum sauce.

3   Cover with the lid, reduce the temperature and cook for 6–8 hours or until tender. Remove the fillets and keep warm. Strain the remaining sauce in the cooking pot into a small pan and boil until slightly reduced. Blend the cornflour with 480 ml of water, stir into the sauce and cook, stirring, until thickened. Slice the fillets, arrange on individual serving plates, drizzle with a little sauce and garnish with the parsley and plums.

4   Serve with freshly cooked noodles and salad.

CHILLI PORK WITH PEANUTS AND PEACHES

SERVES **4**

Good with rice, baked potatoes or in taco shells, this spicy pork and peanut mixture may be hotted up by adding extra chilli, or cooled by cutting it down to a mere pinch.

450 g lean boneless pork, cut into thin strips

1 tsp chilli powder

1 tsp ground allspice

2 garlic cloves, crushed

2 tsp sesame oil

2 tbsp olive oil

1 onion, thinly sliced

50 g roasted peanuts

225 g French beans, lightly cooked

425 g can peach slices, drained

freshly ground black pepper

TO SERVE

250 ml low-fat crème fraîche

1 Place the pork in a dish, then mix in the chilli, allspice, garlic and sesame oil. Cover and leave to marinate for at least 2 hours or overnight in the refrigerator.

2 Heat the oil and stir-fry the onion for 5 minutes before adding the pork. Stir-fry the meat until lightly browned all over. Add the peanuts and cook for a further 2 minutes before mixing in the beans and peaches.

3 Continue cooking for about 5 minutes, so that the beans are piping hot and the pork is cooked through. Add some seasoning to taste, then serve at once, offering low-fat crème fraîche with the spicy pork.

NUTRITIONAL VALUES

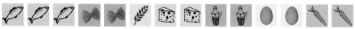

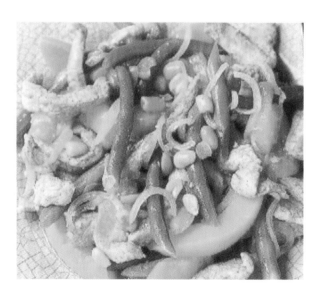

STEAK AND VEGETABLE HOTPOT

SERVES **4**

This is a versatile, flavoursome stew. Keep it very old-fashioned by serving it with mashed, boiled or baked potatoes, or use it as the base for a number of dishes.

NUTRITIONAL VALUES

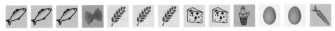

350 g stewing or braising steak, diced

3 tbsp plain flour

freshly ground black pepper

2 tbsp oil

1 large leek, sliced and rinsed

1 large onion, chopped

1 carrot, halved and sliced

1 bay leaf

2 parsley sprigs

1 thyme sprig

600 ml beef stock

2 parsnips, cut into chunks

½ turnip or celery root, peeled and cut into chunks

350 g brussels sprouts, halved unless very small

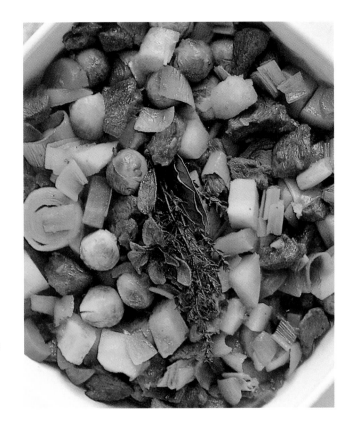

1 The meat should be diced not cut in chunks. Toss it with the flour and plenty of seasoning. Heat the oil, then add the meat and cook it, stirring often, until sealed and lightly browned.

2 Add the leek, onion and carrot, then cook for 5 minutes, stirring. Tie the bay and herb sprigs into a bunch and add it to the pan with the stock. Stir until the liquid is just simmering, then cover tightly and regulate the heat so that the stew simmers very gently: Boiling will toughen the meat. Cook for 2½ hours, stirring occasonally.

3 Add the parsnips and turnip or celery root to the stew, stir well and re-cover. Simmer for 15 minutes, or until the parsnips and turnip or celery root are tender.

4 Taste and adjust the seasoning before serving piping hot.

DESSERTS

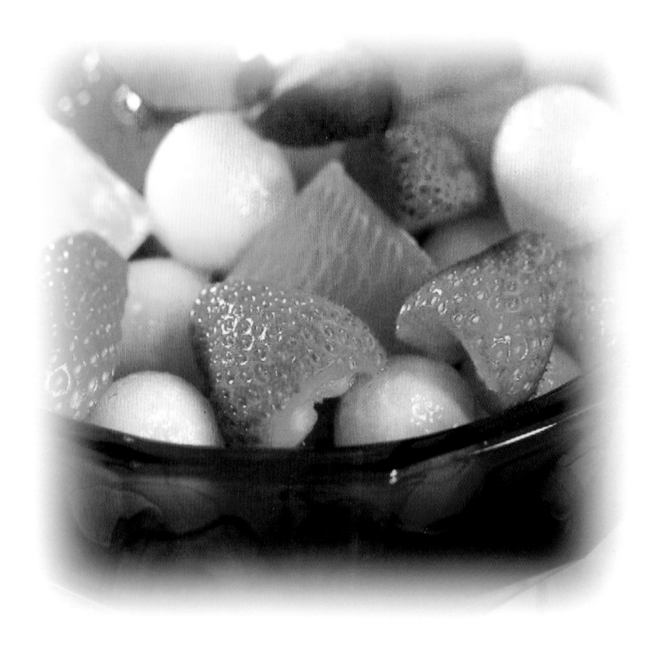

FRUIT CHAAT

SERVES **4**

I am sure you will be suprised to read the list of ingredients: chilli powder and pepper with fruit, in a dessert? Be suprised again when you've tried it and seen for yourself how well it works.

Fruit chaats are very popular at tea parties, dinner parties and other special occasions.

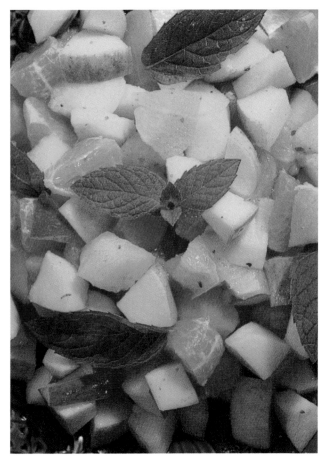

175 g guavas, tinned, drained

175 g honeydew melon

110 g pears

110 g apple

110 g tangerines

1/4 tsp cumin seeds, crushed

pinch of chilli powder

pinch of freshly ground black pepper

2–3 tsp artificial sugar

2 tbsp fresh orange juice

2 tsp lemon juice

TO GARNISH

fresh mint leaves, slightly crushed or broken

NUTRITIONAL VALUES

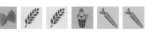

1   Cut up all the fruits into small cubes or tiny segments so that the spices can mingle into the fruits easily.

2   Mix all the spices together in a bowl, pour in the artificial sugar and the orange and lemon juice, stir and shake the mixture to blend them. Pour this over the fruit, mix gently, garnish with the mint leaves and chill well before serving.

WATERMELON WEDGES WITH MANGO-BERRY SALSA

SERVES **6-12**

This is an easy 'throw it together' dessert that your friends will ask you to make again and again. It's low in calories yet deliciously sweet.

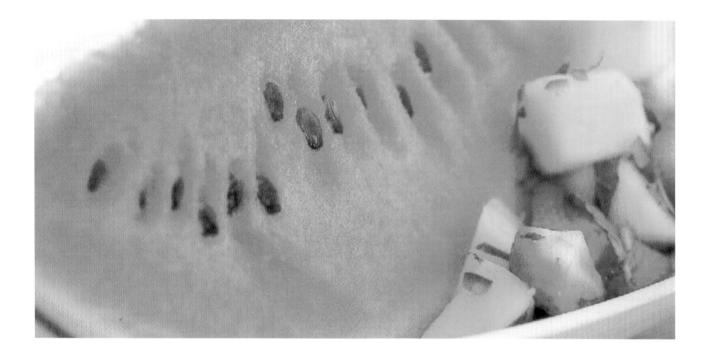

NUTRITIONAL VALUES

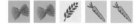

12 x 4 cm thick watermelon wedges

400 g chopped mango

100 g fresh strawberries, hulled and chopped

1 tbsp finely chopped jalapeño chilli

2 tbsp finely chopped fresh mint

2 tbsp honey

1 Combine all the ingredients except the watermelon in a medium bowl. Refrigerate the salsa and watermelon until chilled.

2 To serve, spoon the mango salsa over the watermelon wedges.

STRAWBERRIES WITH MELON AND ORANGE

SERVES **4**

Strawberries and other berry fruits are a good source of fibre, whereas melons – containing so much water and inedible skin – are not so fibre-rich. Mix them together and you have a good combination of flavours and textures, as well as a colourful dessert. Remove the membrane from the orange segments if you prefer.

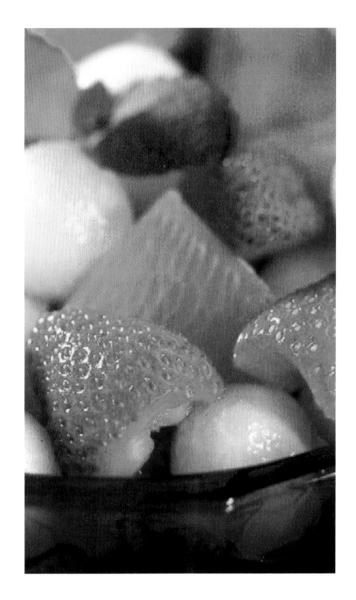

350–450 g halved strawberries

1 small Galia melon, balled

2 oranges

125 g orange juice (optional)

TO GARNISH

mint leaves

1 Place the halved strawberries in a bowl with the melon balls. Peel the oranges and break into segments, then cut them in half or chop them roughly, depending on size.

2 Add the oranges to the other fruits with any juices, adding extra orange juice if necessary. The fruits will usually create their own juice, especially if the melon is ripe.

3 Leave to stand for 30 minutes. Serve the fruit salad at room temperature, decorated with the fresh mint leaves.

NUTRITIONAL VALUES

DAIRY MOULDS

A delicious low-fat version of the French 'coeur a la crème', *this dairy blend makes a light and delightful accompaniment to soft fruits of all kinds. It is also good with fresh dates or figs, or drizzled with honey and sprinkled with nuts.*

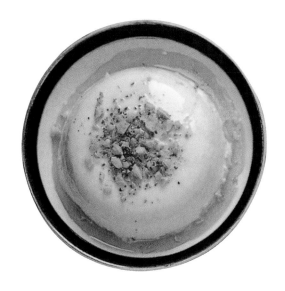

450 g low-fat cottage cheese

150 ml plain low-fat yoghurt

150 ml low-fat crème fraîche

3 tbsp warm water

1 sachet powdered gelatine, about 11 g

NUTRITIONAL VALUES

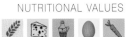

1 Sieve the cottage cheese into a bowl. Beat in the yoghurt and low-fat crème fraîche.

2 Pour the water into a small bowl, sprinkle on the gelatine, stir well and stand the bowl in a pan of warm water. Leave for about 5 minutes for the gelatine to dissolve. Pour the gelatine mixture into the cheese and beat well.

3 Spoon the cheese into 6 individual moulds. Heart-shaped ones are traditional, or you can improvise by using ramekin dishes or yoghurt pots covered with muslin and inverted. Stand the moulds on a wire rack over a plate and leave them to drain in the refrigerator overnight.

4 Turn out the moulds and serve the cheese well chilled.

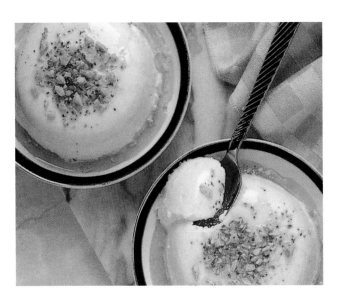

BANANA CUSTARD

SERVES **3 – 4**

This is a tasty and refreshing end to a meal, or can be served as a summer treat!

NUTRITIONAL VALUES

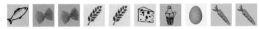

2 bananas, sliced

shredded rind and juice of 1 lemon

750 ml low-fat créme fraîche or low-fat yoghurt

75 g pecans, chopped roughly

1 tbsp honey

75 g bran

skimmed milk

1   Toss banana slices in lemon juice, then place in a bowl. Carefully mix in low-fat crème fraîche or the low-fat yoghurt, nuts, honey and bran.

2   If the mixture is very thick, add 1 or 2 tbsp of skimmed milk to thin it down.

3   Decorate with lemon rind just before serving.

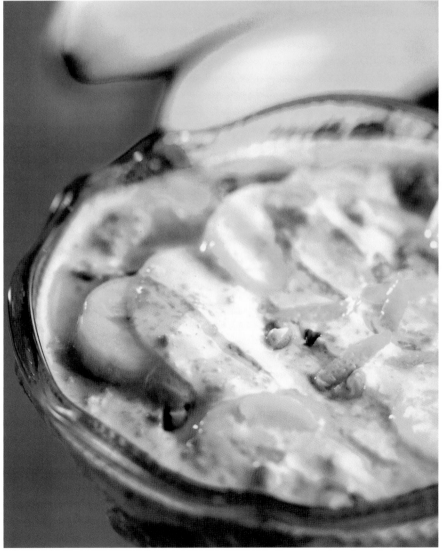

OATY BISCUITS

MAKES **12**

A very high fibre and tasty snack to accompany a cup of tea or coffee, to be had with breakfast, lunch or in between!

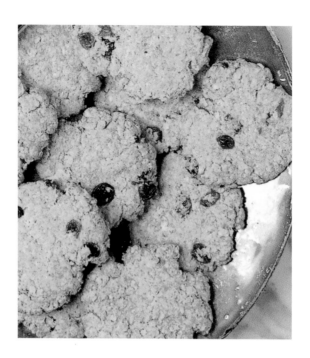

60 g wholewheat flour

½ tsp baking soda

187 g oatmeal

grated peel and juice of 1 orange

50 g golden raisins

4 tbsp oil

3 tbsp unsweetened apple juice

1 Preheat the oven at 180°C/gas mark 4, and grease a baking sheet.

2 Mix the flour, baking soda, oats, orange peel and golden raisins. Mix in the oil and orange juice with enough apple juice to make a firm dough.

3 Turn the dough out onto a floured surface and knead it lightly, then divide it in half and cut each half into 6 equal portions. Flatten each portion into a 3–6 cm circle.

4 Place the biscuits on the baking sheet as they are shaped, and bake for 15–20 minutes, until browned. Transfer the biscuits to a wire rack to cool.

NUTRITIONAL VALUES

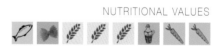

FRUIT SALAD

SERVES **4**

Lovely and colourful, with a hint of tropical flavour. Needless to say, all the fruit must be as fresh as possible, but if you cannot obtain fresh blueberries, use frozen ones instead.

2 medium-sized juicy oranges

2 limes

30 g raspberries

30 g golden raspberries

30 g strawberries

30 g blueberries

30 g blackberries

1 large papaya

2 kiwi fruit, peeled and sliced

20 g fresh coconut meat,
    shredded, or 25 g
    desiccated coconut

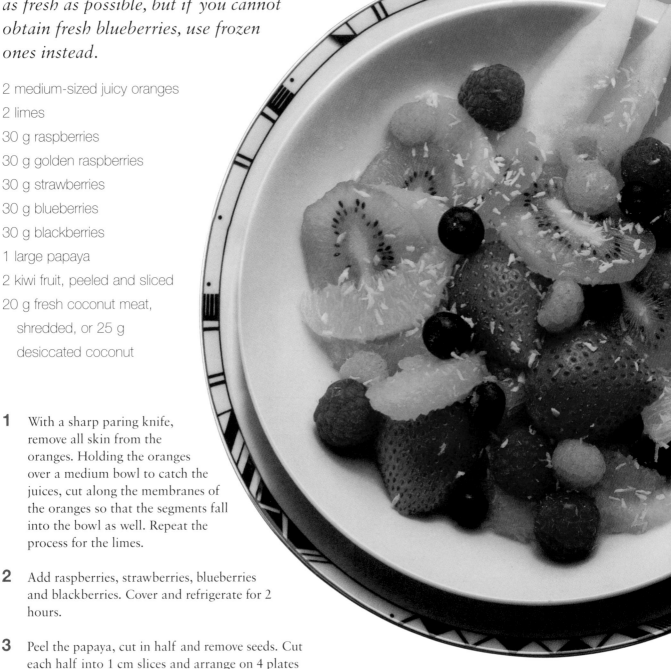

1   With a sharp paring knife, remove all skin from the oranges. Holding the oranges over a medium bowl to catch the juices, cut along the membranes of the oranges so that the segments fall into the bowl as well. Repeat the process for the limes.

2   Add raspberries, strawberries, blueberries and blackberries. Cover and refrigerate for 2 hours.

3   Peel the papaya, cut in half and remove seeds. Cut each half into 1 cm slices and arrange on 4 plates with the sliced kiwi fruit.

4   Spoon the berry and orange mixture, with the juices, over the papaya. Sprinkle with coconut.

NUTRITIONAL VALUES

PRUNE AND NUT QUICK BREAD

MAKES **10** SLICES

Other dried fruit may be used in place of prunes – raisins or golden raisins are good,
or simply add a little mixed dried fruit.

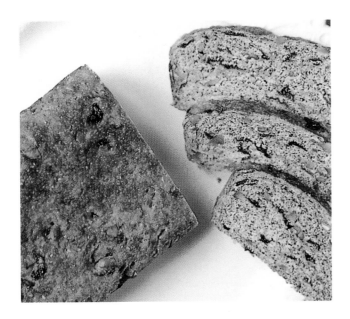

250 g hard wholewheat flour

2 tbsp margarine

50 g pitted and chopped ready-to-eat prunes

75 g finely chopped walnuts

167 ml milk

1 envelope active-dried yeast

1   Place the flour in a bowl. Cut in the margarine, then stir in the prunes and walnuts. Heat the milk until it is hand hot – if it gets any hotter, leave it to cool before adding the yeast. Stir in the yeast and leave for about 15 minutes until frothy.

2   Make a well in the dry ingredients, then add the milk and yeast and gradually mix it into the ingredients to make a firm dough. Add an extra few drops of milk if necessary to bind the ingredients but not to make the dough sticky.

3   Grease a 450 g bread tin with 450 ml capacity. Turn the dough out on a lightly floured surface and knead it thoroughly for 10 minutes, until smooth and elastic. Press stray nuts back into the dough as you knead it. Place the dough in the pan, pressing it down into the corners. Cover the top loosely with oiled plastic wrap and leave the dough in a warm place until risen in a dome above the rim of the tin – this can take up to a couple of hours depending on the heat of the dough and the room.

4   Preheat the oven to 220°C/gas mark 7.

5   Brush the loaf with a little warm water, then bake it for 35–40 minutes, until browned on top. Turn the loaf out and tap its base – it should produce a hollow sound when the bread is cooked. Cool on a wire rack. Serve sliced, and if required, spread thinly with a low-fat spread.

NUTRITIONAL VALUES

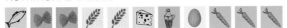

EASY PINWHEEL BUNS

MAKES **9**

These are a useful cook's cheat, making use of bread mix instead of weighing and preparing a traditional dough. If you need the extra fibre to balance the content of other meals, you can use a wholewheat bread mix, but the results are not so pleasing.

150 g dried mixed fruit

167 ml unsweetened apple juice

275 g package bread mix

250 ml milk, warmed

a little flour

1 tsp ground cinnamon

NUTRITIONAL VALUES

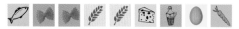

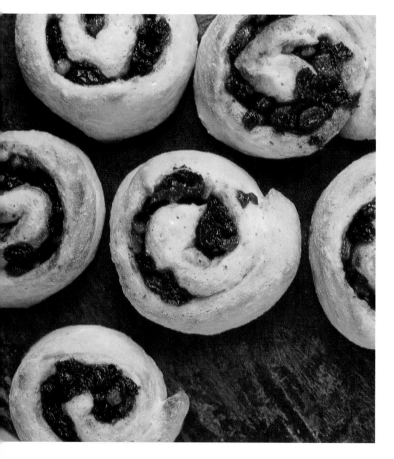

1. Place the fruit in a saucepan with the apple juice and bring to a boil. Reduce the heat and simmer for 10 minutes, or until the juice has evaporated, shaking the pan frequently towards the end of cooking to avoid burning. Set aside to cool slightly.

2. Grease a 22.5 cm square pan.

3. Make up the bread mix following the package instructions, using the milk instead of water. Knead the dough until smooth and elastic, then roll it out on a lightly floured surface into a 22.5–25 cm square.

4. Mix the cinnamon into the fruit, then spread it over the dough, leaving a clear gap all around the edge. Dampen the edges of the dough. roll uo the dough from one side, like a swiss roll.

5. Use a sharp knife to cut the roll into nine even slices, then place these, cut sides up, in the greased tin. Cover loosely with oiled plastic and leave in a warm place until well risen – the dough should be doubled in thickness and this will take some considerable time.

6. Meanwhile, preheat the oven at 220°C/gas mark 7.

7. Bake the rolls for 20–30 minutes, until browned and firm. Allow to cool in the baking tin for 15 minutes, then transfer them to a wire rack.

8. The pinwheels are delicious served warm.

APPLE AND CARROT CAKE

MAKES **16 SLICES**

This is moist, well flavoured and healthy dessert.

250 g self-raising wholewheat flour

125 g margerine

1 tsp cinnamon

150 g chopped walnuts

100 g raisins

300 g peeled, cored and grated dessert apples

150 g grated carrot

grated peel of 1 orange

2 large eggs

4 tbsp fresh orange juice

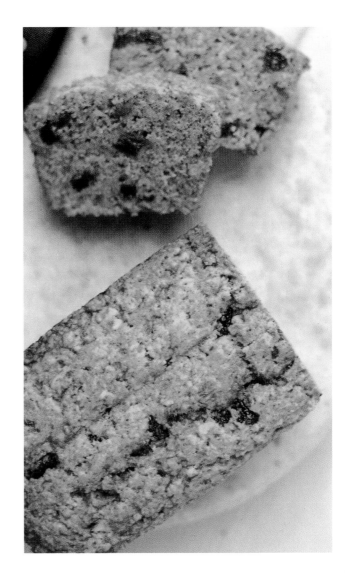

1   Line the base and grease a loaf tin with 1 l capacity.

2   Preheat the oven to 180°C/gas mark 4.

3   Place the flour in a bowl and mix well, then cut in the margarine and stir in the cinnamon. Stir in the walnuts, raisins, apples and carrot. Add the orange peel, eggs and juice, then beat well until thoroughly combined.

4   Spoon the mixture into the prepared pan, smooth the top and bake for about 1¼ hours, or until the cake is well risen and firm to the touch. Turn out and cool on a wire rack.

NUTRITIONAL VALUES

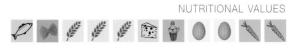

INDEX

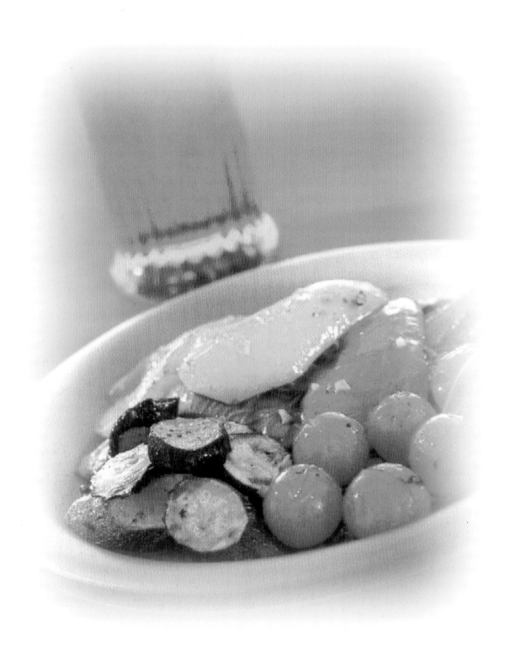